The Light at the End of the Refrigerator

Foods That Heal
Spa Cooking

by
MAUREEN KENNEDY
SALAMAN

M.K.S., Inc.

Published by
M.K.S., Inc.
1259 El Camino Real, Suite 1500
Menlo Park, CA 94025
Telephone: (415) 854-9355
FAX: (415) 854-9292

Produced by:
Julia Bauer
DEW Communications
Sacramento, CA

Cover Design by:
Mark Simpson
Simpson Communications
Palm Harbor, FL

■ ISBN: 0-913087-165
Library of Congress Card No. 89-051450

INTRODUCTION

Just throw it away!! Empty your refrigerator NOW of all that processed sugar, artificial fat and any ingredient you can't pronounce. Some of the stuff way in the back is probably old enough to vote, and has expiration dates written in "B.C." - which in this case means *before coagulation.*

Good job! Now that it is as empty as the U.S. Treasury, I can help you see the light at the end of the refrigerator.

Most of us have been brainwashed into seeing unhealthful food as adequate diets to live by. We eat to entertain our taste buds, then we suffer the torments of migraines, allergies and heart disease, with not a clue as to the dietary connection.

What I'm about to tell you comes from experience, believe me! My eating habits used to be horrendous! Burger King should have knighted me. Sara Lee was my patron saint.

I entertained my taste buds with fat and sugar, treating my upper gastrointestinal tract as if it were a stainless steel pipe emptying into a garbage disposal. My idea of vigorous exercise was eating faster.

My purpose in writing this cookbook is to show you how you can eat well, and eat right, using certain foods, meals and menus to target ailments, illnesses and injuries.

What you eat is very important to your health, I can't emphasize this enough. However, not everyone reacts the same to the same food. Listen to your body after you've eaten. What is it saying to you? Does it say, "let's go jogging!" Or does it say "I don't want to move for a century." If your meals make you feel slow and sluggish, you're probably due for a change.

If you also came to this book to break free of food addictions and then plan your loved ones' escape, you've come to the right place. It sounds like a cliche, but it's true: It's not how much you eat, it's *how* you eat.

I was in this regimental rut for years. My idea of a good diet was eating less of the bad stuff.

I was determined to get unhooked, but no matter how resolute I was, somehow the thought of not seeing a twinkie for an entire week seemed like the violation of a natural law. The law of cavity.

Living in the fast lane, I raced in and out of fast food restaurants. I thought I was personally responsible for adding another billion to the McDonald's sign, but pretty soon I wouldn't have been able to fit through the golden arches. I was even known for running into a burning restaurant to save the dessert cart.

I tried to diet - I really did! It was the worst three hours of my life.

I saw myself in the mirror - too much of me - and became determined to change, not only for my sake, but for my husband's and children's. After all, a role model shouldn't display too many rolls in the midsection.

Finally, I broke the habit of bad taste. When I tried to cheat, and bit into a glazed donut, it tasted like a mouthful of lard. Hamburgers tasted like shredded rubber surrounded by wet tissue. I even took down my shrine to Sara Lee: I gave away my cookie jar.

My next step was to plan my family's escape.

My husband was not a firm believer in exercise. You might say he was a flabby believer in loafing. He thought - and he even said this! - that the earth rotating around the sun was enough exercise for him.

The only way I could get him to do deep knee bends was to put the TV remote control between his toes. He was at the age where his knees buckled but his belt wouldn't.

While he didn't seem to mind growing old, his body wasn't taking it well. The children used to rub his tummy for good luck.

And he wasn't getting any younger. He and our house suffered from the same problems: a thinning roof, sagging foundation and clogged pipes. I used to remind him of the high cost of funerals.

My daughter was calorie conscious. When she was conscious, she was eating calories. She tried to diet, but her idea of a continental breakfast was eating a continent. She definitely had a weight problem - she couldn't wait for the next feeding.

When I told her she should get into shape, she said, "Round is a shape." I tried patiently to explain to her that food is the fuel your body burns, giving off heat, which is measured in calories. She quipped, "So my body is basically a pot-bellied stove."

She wasn't the only one to be thoughtless. Once when we were shopping she asked me if I thought her choice of dresses made her look fat. I said, "No, it's your thighs that make you look fat."

She saved me approximately $100,000. I didn't have to send her to college, she already knew everything.

My teenage son thought his acne was caused by the caffeine in the six pack of Coke he drank every day. So he switched to Pepsi. I told him brewer's yeast, which is high in zinc, is what he needed. So he switched to beer. Wrong again!

The project I was taking on was not going to be easy. People who say "nothing is impossible" never had teenage kids. My children were two siblings who each should have been an only child.

I figured out why my teenagers grew so fast. It was all that fast food. They believed the four basic food groups were: McDonalds, Burger King, Taco Bell and Wendy's.

They thought catsup was pureed tomato, and it was the only vegetable they ate on a regular basis. They became ugly at the mention of the word "carrot." And if I served them a salad, I could prepare to grow old waiting for them to eat it.

My motive for trying to convert them was selfless mother love. I saw myself as Mother Theresa. They saw me as the queen of mean, Leona Helmsley.

One of the lessons I try to teach my children throughout their lives is that nothing is useless, even if it simply serves as a bad example. Even a stopped clock is right twice a day! Keeping this principle in mind, my daughter took my first loaf of homemade whole grain bread and used it as a doorstop.

Luckily for me, my family put cooking on par with mud wrestling, and I was the only one accorded the privilege. So they had no choice but to eat what I fed them.

At first we ate sparingly, like the occupants of a lifeboat cast adrift on the lonely sea. I knew that this was necessary to throw off the poisons accumulated through years of poor eating habits. I began to feel we were on a lifeboat too, especially when, during the holidays, neighbors and friends good intentionally brought us cookies and cakes. As I shoveled the "goodies" into the garbage disposal, my husband reminded me of the starving children in Africa. I told him they'd still be starving if they ate this stuff.

I have to admit, my cooking could've tasted better. I've since learned the secret to flavoring with herbs and making natural foods taste succulent, but back then it was a well-kept secret I had yet to find out. I believed, like many others, that healthy food couldn't taste good.

After one particularly high fiber dinner, my son requested his beverage be fabric softener.

I was fighting tradition. I was fighting the wholesome, all-American family depicted on billboards who routinely ate bacon for breakfast, hamburgers for lunch and pizza for dinner.

One morning my sleepy-eyed, bacon-and-eggs oriented son came to breakfast muttering something about weird eating habits upsetting the food chain. He suggested I scatter his meals over the lawn and let him graze.

My daughter came to dinner with a feedbag strapped to her head. I told her to quit horsing around and clean her stall.

My husband rose to my defense. He said, "Don't be so hard on your mother. She's just learning a new skill."

My response was somewhat less than kind. "You are out of my will," I said between clenched teeth.

It would have been easier to cook for the Manson family. Each night at the dinner table I felt like the defendant in a murder case facing the jury.

My husband was certain that eating so many natural foods would cause him to die of natural causes.

My mother-in-law, as usual, proved whose side she was on. The punishment for bigamy, by the way, is two mother-in-laws. Instructed by her doctor to take her medications with food, she suggested all my cooking should be taken with medication.

Even our household pet, Happy Cat, turned up her nose up at my food, and then at me. She would sit for hours glaring at the leftovers I put in her dish as though waiting for the wine list.

But I was determined that super-nutrition would prevail. It was going to be whole wheat and nothing but the wheat, so help me God.

My cooking improved as I began to accept substitutes. I learned to substitute real food: whole grains, honey, and fresh raw vegetables and fruit for refined white flour, processed sugar, and canned vegetables and fruit. I created recipes substituting concentrated fruit juices for sugar and dried fruits instead of chocolate chips.

As I saw my son's acne clear up, and my husband and daughter lose weight, they began to compliment me on my meals instead of criticize. My son learned that brewer's yeast is not beer and didn't mind when I added it to his daily fruit smoothie. And the twigs and leaves jokes stopped.

In fact, the long-running debate with my family over healthy living served me well. In attempting to find scientific studies to convince them of the nutrition answer, I gathered more and more information.

A newsletter I started for an alternative doctor who was facing court charges for helping a multitude of people (including a cherished friend) became successful and I went on to edit three other health publications.

I found myself leading the way as the health and fitness industry grew. I was asked to do a radio show which soon became the most listened to nutrition talk show in Northern California.

I learned that nutrition not only helps maintain good overall health, but is used by alternative medical practitioners to cure illnesses and ailments. My family and I were entirely convinced when my husband nearly lost his right hand to infection and a heavy intake of vitamin C dramatically cured it - after the only hope orthodox medicine offered was amputation.

I began to gather a large database of research on natural healing, as much to continue the conversion of my family and friends as the outer world in general.

Figuring people would be hungry for nutritional enlightenment, I began lecturing - mostly to myself. I guess at the time potential listeners were on a starvation diet.

Things were different when I first started lecturing on the value of health food over 20 years ago. In those days people thought of health food "nuts" as strange iconoclasts from Vegetaria.

I'd always enjoyed writing. It was a gift God gave me. I was only eight years old when I had my first article published in a children's magazine. After losing a dear friend to cancer I took the pain and passion of the experience and infused it onto paper. The result was the 1983 release of my first book, *Nutrition - the Cancer Answer*.

In 1989 it was voted the best health book by the *American Book Exchange* and is now an international best seller.

My second book, *The Diet Bible*, arose from my success at weight loss, and what I learned to maintain a high level of wellness.

I traveled the world gathering nutritional information. I went to Egypt, Turkey, the United Kingdom, Canada, Japan and Australia, just to name a few countries. I lived with the Masai of East Africa in a little dung hut with a dirt floor. I volunteered with the National Health Federation, editing their magazine.

Foods that Heal was my third book, and was embraced with great enthusiasm by millions of people whose lives were changed by the simple, natural, but effective answers they found. It is a reader-friendly guide through the medical alphabet of ailments from acne to wrinkles.

Since then, many have tried to imitate it, but these counterfeit books give only superficial palliatives, while *Foods That Heal* stands alone, rooting out the cause of ailments.

As a result of being interviewed on television with *Cancer Answer*, the station asked me to do my own television show, which is now on satellite airing all over the world, and is in its eighth year. Today, I put in 100 hours a month doing television guest appearances, plus my own show.

All my books have become best-sellers, and I do regular book signings around the country. At my most recent book signing, over 1,000 people jammed the shopping center, and the police had to come for crowd control. The fire department declared me a fire hazard because people were jamming the doorways, creating traffic hazards. I asked them for a certificate.

I'm grateful to God and to all the many individuals who are responsible for my success. I'm also grateful *for* them, as I know this knowledge will benefit all who learn of it.

Today, health food is not a craze, it's a business. In fact, people put so much stock in it, the FDA (some call it the Faster Death Association) is getting in on the act. Unfortunately, because it functions as a protection racket for the drug industry, it's been as great an asset to the health food industry as mud wrestling has been to the performing arts.

As explained in my book *Nutrition, The Cancer Answer*, because of the thalidomide scare, the Harris-Kefauver amendment of 1962 gave the FDA the responsibility to pass or fail any new drug, but didn't rule on efficacy. Since then, a deadly log jam has been created by the FDA which is costing by far more lives than it is saving.

We all want our drugs to be efficacious, but who is better able to judge? The doctor who works closely with his patients and will lose his patients and his livelihood if he continues to use a drug that doesn't work, or a third party bureaucrat in Washington, D.C.?

The trouble with government agencies like the FDA is there is no citizen control, so it enjoys the same kind of tyrannical power over you as an oriental potentate. The FDA is an unelected unconstitutional unresponsive fourth branch of the federal government. Like all government agencies, the FDA functions like the alimentary canal of a baby - with a voracious appetite at one end and no sense of responsibility at the other.

Have you ever noticed when your cup runneth over, someone knocketh your elbow?

Despite the popularity of health and nutrition, it remains an uphill battle. You still have to ask for no MSG, and it's like the food service establishment doesn't know the meaning of the term "natural state," or they think vegetables come out of the ground batter-dipped and fried. You don't want to know what they put into your gravy, or your beef for that matter.

Despite the stress and difficulties, I love what I do and who I am. I love the people I know and meet. I consider my work an anointing straight from the Heavenly Father.

One of the most gratifying blessings I received from God came from the mouth of babes: my son. He didn't know I was listening when someone asked him what he thought of my new-found success. He said, "It just proves to me the scripture that says, `He that is servant among you will be master of all.' "

This is and always has been my principle: to serve God by serving people. The bible says when you plant a seed, you will be overcome with blessing. As a result, the seed that leaves your hand never leaves your life; it's just planted into your future.

I set about to always serve and blessings come back to me. I don't sell products, I solve problems. I adhere to the Christian point of view that you always retain the heart of a servant. First you bless others, then you are so blessed. You don't have to look for blessings, they just come.

"Give and it shall be given unto you; good measure, pressed down and shaken together, and running over, shall men give unto your bosom. For with the same measure that ye meter it shall be measured to you again." - Luke 6:38

When I saw the multitude of blessings that came out of Christian television; the lives saved, kids gotten off drugs, families brought back together and lost people brought back through the knowledge of Christ, I wanted my work's profits to support this most honorable medium. I'm happy to report my work is raising several million dollars a year to sustain a multitude of independent Christian stations. I am viewed and listened to by millions of people around the world.

Now I bring you *The Light at the End of the Refrigerator*, a companion cookbook to *Foods That Heal* for your culinary pleasure and nutritional needs; and I hope a few laughs as well.

In my effort to bring both my family and yours life-perpetuating foods that don't taste like kitty litter, but instead are succulent, delicious and easy to prepare, I've compiled these recipes. My family eats these dishes with relish, (they used to use ketchup, mayonnaise and sugar) as long as I don't tell them how healthful they are. I hope yours will too.

Many of these recipes are original - you'll find them nowhere else. They have been kitchen-tested, to be sure they aren't complicated. And they are delicious - I should know, since most have been taste-tested by me! We've designed them so they shouldn't take you more than one hour to create and are inexpensive to prepare. They were designed to save you time, money, and even your life and health. No expense has been spared to make these recipes as economical as possible.

You're now entering an adventurous new world of healing with meals. Using the dynamics of food nutrition, you can make a difference in how you feel and how you heal.

Consider the principles I've outlined in each chapter, try the recipes, and get creative! Even the Betty Crocker cookbook has a list of the nutrients contained in foods. Once you know what to look for, the supermarket is your healing clinic! Let this book serve as your guiding light to good food, good health and a good life.

Lovingly,
Maureen Kennedy Salaman

To My Precious Friend, Karl Heinz Rolfes

A masterpiece within a masterpiece is each recipe in this book full of them created by Karl Rolfes. Somehow, mere expressions on paper cannot fully transmit my gratitude to him. It is as if my words need spiritual vitamins and minerals to attain the power and poetry imprisoned within me.

The wonder of it all is that Karl's greatest career achievements are in fields of art outside of gourmet cooking. However, through the years, he has experimented and perfected recipes in his kitchens, doing what he loves and loving what he does, aiming for and reaching the Mount Everest level of quality. Every time Karl chefs for my parties, I receive rave reviews.

Although the quality and novelty of his creations would warrant his presiding over the kitchen of a five star restaurant, Karl, by profession, is a master hair designer, trained for seven years in this art in Germany. Before coming to the United States, he coiffed the fairest heads in the film industry in his native land as well as models posing for the German version of Vogue magazine.

Visiting New York briefly, he was invited to join the hair stylists at Kenneth's, the "in" beauty studio of Manhattan celebrities, but decided, instead, to move on. Then he made a mistake - a happy one for himself and me: he stopped off to see San Francisco on his way to Australia. He and his heart decided to stay for good.

There should be a special kind of award for Karl's cooking, which is as decorative as it is savory and nutritious. His dishes help me stay trim, lean and energy-charged. After years of enjoying his creative cookery, I feel selfish in not having shared his recipes earlier. However, that was not an intentional sin. Let me compensate for this now by inviting you into the pages of this book and into a new adventure in eating for brimming-over good health, for well-being and for fun, too!

ACKNOWLEDGEMENTS

My acknowledgements start gratefully with Dr. Ross Gordon, whose healing brilliance is so rare and real that without him I would not have walked away from a serious injury. He helped me to be more myself, more the person God intended me to be, and it is possible that without him I would never have recognized myself, or grown to be what it is in me to be.

I point with pride to the commitment, loyalty and assiduousness of my staff. For them, selfishness and personal glory are subordinated to team effort and team glory. The success I have achieved as an individual has been because I am a part of this dedicated team.

To the officers, Board members, staff, and membership of the National Health Federation: I have served them with passion and dedication for over two decades, and for the last ten years as their President. May God continue to make them brave and keep them true.

Many think of fulfillment as something to be found in money, wealth, success and applause; and don't learn until it's too late that the greatest gift God gives is loving friends. In this I am the wealthiest of people. My true riches are manifest in the following people. They are, each and every one, my life's greatest treasure: Lia Belli, Charlet Blachbourn, Norma and Russ Bixler, Freda and Claude Bowers, Fran and Don Braca, Alicia and Red Buttons, Jane and Aldo Fontana, Bobbie and Tony Corteze, Betsy Dohrman, Jo Ann Dupont, Dehlia Erlick, Bella Farrow, Shirley and Kenny Foreman, Kurt Foreman, Kenny Foreman, Jr., Blackie Gonzales, Dr. Gary Gordon, Kathryn Grayson, Jeffrey Harsh, Cory and Michael Haskett, Connie and Ron Haus, Vonda Haus, Fred Hirth, William Holloway, Nancy and Jack Horton, Wendy and Frank Jordan, Dr. Hans Kugler, Margaret and Dean Lesher, Irsula Marston, Ruth and Merl McAnich, Anne and Jim Regal, Karl Rolfes, Michael Rosenfield, Fran Sanchez, Jim Scheer, Dee and Glenn Simmons, Phil Sinclair, Jo Ann and Jim Thompson, Cynthia and Mark Thornberg, Karen and Scott Tips, and Holly and Jonathan Wright.

TABLE OF CONTENTS

THE LIGHT

God gave us the ingredients. It's up to us to make the bread.

The menus that accompany each chapter in this book are based on an age-old principle: eat like a king at breakfast, like a prince at lunch, and like a pauper at dinner. Eat brunch like a duke! Well, anyway, you get the idea. These are wise words, as they have our good health, well-being and weight control in mind.

Avoid eating a lot of food before bedtime; it stresses the body, and especially the heart. In fact, most heart attacks occur in the wee hours of the morning, during sleep time. Large amounts of heavy foods can also contribute to sleeplessness.

It was the wise John W. Gardner who said, "All happiness depends upon a leisurely breakfast." Taking your time to eat not only helps your outlook, but your stomach as well.

You'll see breakfast recipes here that aren't what you usually expect. That's because it's important to eat filling, hearty foods to get an energetic start to the day. Complex carbohydrates, like beans and lentils, fill this need very well. Cakes and breads that contain whole grains work too. Stretch your horizons! Remember, the only difference between a rut and the grave is the depth.

Consider these principles of good eating when looking at these menus. Some chapters/ailments relate to each other, so more than one may apply to your particular problem. And if the food doesn't do it, the humor may. Remember, laughter maketh merry medicine.

CHAPTER 1
Acne

If your skin resembles the moon's surface, consider these zinc-rich recipes to stamp out your acne. And remember, lots of water will wash those pores clean of the oils that clog them and lead to pimples.

Many, many people have come to me to give me success stories about how they cleared their skin with zinc and zinc-rich foods. Now I'm passing the secret on to you.

When someone gives you some nonsense about your looks not being important, consider these humorous words by Jean Kerr: "I'm tired of all this nonsense about beauty being only skin-deep. That's deep enough. What do you want, an adorable pancreas?"

BREAKFAST

BUCKWHEAT AND WALNUT PANCAKES

1 cup buckwheat	1 cup soda water
1/4 cup chopped walnuts	

Mix ingredients and stir well. Add blueberry or honey, if desired. Let thicken for ten minutes. Heat pan with butter or olive oil. Make small patties with batter, and let slightly brown on both sides. Serve with pure maple syrup or fresh fruit.

LUNCH

MEAT VEGETABLE LOAF

1 lb. ground chuck	1/2 clove garlic, chopped
2 egg yolks, beaten	1/2 tsp. parsley
1 medium onion, chopped	1/4 tsp. oregano
4 carrots, chopped	1/8 tsp. black pepper
4 stalks celery, chopped	1/8 tsp. nutmeg
4 small tomatoes, chopped	1/8 tsp. rosemary

Mix together: beef, eggs, onion, carrots, celery, parsley, tomato and garlic. Add

2

spices. Blend well and place in loaf pan. Bake in 350 degree oven 45 minutes to an hour or until meat has cooked through and top is brown.

DINNER

TABBOULEH

1/2 cup bulgur
1 small onion, finely chopped
1 green onion, finely chopped
1/2 cup chopped fresh parsley or 1/4 cup dried
1/3 cup lemon juice
3 tbsp. fresh mint leaves or 3 tsp. dried
1/4 cup olive oil
3-4 tomatoes, cut in wedges

Soak bulgur in cold water to cover 30 minutes. Drain, place bulgur on a cloth and wring out excess water. Mix the onion, green onion, parsley and lemon juice together. Toss with the bulgur. Refrigerate at least 1/2 hour. Add mint to olive oil. Mix with bulgur mixture just before serving.

To serve, mound the bulgur on a plate and garnish with tomato wedges. If preferred, the tomatoes can be chopped fine and added to the bulgur mixture. Serves four.

CHAPTER 2
Addictions

If you think you can get away with living in the fast lane, be warned. You may get to the exit ramp a lot quicker.

If temptation tries you, think on this most quoted of Biblical scriptures and be strong for Him and you.

My grace is sufficient for thee. My strength is made perfect in weakness. - 2 Corinthians 12:9

The following recipes contain foods helpful in alleviating the stress, depression and withdrawal symptoms associated with kicking an addiction. Lentils, in particular, are excellent depression relievers. They work to stabilize the blood sugar, an underlying cause of addiction when it leads to depression. Cook up a big pot once a week, divide it into serving sizes and freeze it. For breakfast, take out a bag and heat it up. Add some alfalfa sprouts for tryptophan and folic acid, nature's relaxant and anti-depressant. While "on the wagon," eat healthy, and you'll find you feel much better about being on the road to recovery.

Those who think they are in the groove are usually in a rut. And remember, the only difference between a rut and the grave is the depth!

BREAKFAST

LENTILS AND HARD BOILED EGGS

4 tbsp. olive oil	2-1/2 cups lentils
1 large onion, chopped	2-1/2 cups beef stock
2 carrots, sliced	1 ham bone
1 celery stalk, chopped	freshly ground pepper
2 cloves garlic, finely chopped	1/4 cup chopped parsley
6 hard boiled eggs, peeled and halved lengthwise	

Heat oil in large, heavy skillet. Add chopped onion, carrots, celery and garlic. Cook over medium heat 5 to 10 minutes until onion is tender and slightly golden.

4

Add lentils and stir. Add stock, covering lentils with 1-1/2" of water left on top. Add ham bone and pepper to taste. Bring to a boil, lower heat and simmer, uncovered, 20-25 minutes or until lentils are soft and there is almost no liquid left. Remove bone. Pour lentils into serving dish; arrange eggs on top. Garnish with parsley.

EGYPTIAN FISH

> 6 medium perch or other firm-fleshed white fish
> sea salt
> pepper
> 2 tbsp. vinegar
> 3 tbsp. chopped parsley
> 1 tbsp. whole wheat bread crumbs
> 1/4 cup olive oil
> 2 medium onions, sliced
> 2 cloves garlic, chopped
> 1/2 cup tahini

Score fish on both sides, salt and pepper to taste and sprinkle with one tablespoon vinegar. Oil 13" x 9" baking pan and preheat oven to 400 degrees. Mix two tablespoons parsley with bread crumbs and sprinkle over baking pan. In skillet, gently fry fish in 3 tablespoons oil until golden on both sides. Reserve oil. Place fish in prepared baking pan. In reserved oil, saute onion slices two minutes. Add garlic and continue sauteing two minutes, or until garlic is golden. Add remaining vinegar, oil and tahini. Mix well. Spoon over fish. Bake 15 minutes. Garnish with remaining parsley.

LUNCH

STUFFED CHICKEN BREAST

4 chicken breasts	juice of 1/2 lemon
1/2 lb. swiss chard or spinach	1 cup sour cream
1/2 medium onion or shallots, chopped	1/8 tsp. black pepper
1/4 tsp. brewer's yeast	1/2 tsp. oregano
1 tsp. parsley	1/8 tsp. nutmeg

Cut chicken breast into a pocket. Stuff pocket with mixture of swiss chard or spinach, chopped onions or shallots, nutmeg, pepper, parsley and yeast. Close pocket with wooden toothpicks. Brown both sides in buttered pan.
Sauce: Mix lemon juice, sour cream, oregano, more parsley and a little more nutmeg. Pour sauce over chicken and pasta of choice.

EGGPLANT PARMESAN

2 eggplants, peeled and sliced	3 sprigs fresh basil or 1 tsp. dry basil
olive oil	1/2 cup grated parmesan cheese
1 tbsp. olive oil	1/4 lb. mozzarella cheese, grated
1 onion, chopped	4 tbsp. soy granules
3 ripe tomatoes, peeled and chopped	

Cook eggplant in olive oil until golden brown. Set aside and keep warm. Preheat oven to 350 degrees. Heat olive oil and briefly saute onion. Add tomatoes and basil. Simmer on low heat about ten minutes. Set aside. Oil a 13" x 9" baking dish. Line the bottom with layer of eggplant. Spread on tomato sauce and sprinkle with cheeses and soy granules. Create two more layers of eggplant, tomato sauce and cheese. The top layer will be cheese. Bake about 40 minutes, or until cheese is bubbly. Serves 6.

DINNER

GAZPACHO

6 large fresh tomatoes, divided	1 tbsp. olive oil
1 large cucumber, halved	1 chili pepper
1 large onion, halved	kelp to taste
1 green bell pepper, halved	1 clove garlic, pressed
1 two-ounce can of pimentos, drained	vegetable seasoning
1/4 cup apple cider vinegar	2.25 oz. can sliced black olives

Put five tomatoes in blender or food processor and puree to make about 18 to 20 ounces. Cut half of the onion, cucumber and pepper into cubes and add to the blender. Blend. Add pimento, kelp, garlic, seasoning, oil and vinegar. Puree. Chill at least three hours.

Serving: Finely chop the remaining ingredients: tomato, onion, pepper, olives and cucumber and sprinkle over bowls of chilled gazbacho.

RAISIN LAMB

1 3-4 lb. lamb breast, trimmed of excess fat.

stuffing:	
1-1/2 cups cooked millet	1 tbsp. black cumin seed
1-1/2 cups cooked lentils	1 tsp. marjoram
1 tbsp. fresh or 1 tsp. dried thyme leaves	1 tsp. parsley
1 tbsp. fresh or 1 tsp. dried mint leaves	sea salt to taste

raisin sauce:
1 cup raisins, soaked overnight in grape juice to cover
1/2 cup unsweetened apricot jam
lemon juice or vinegar to taste

Preheat oven to 400 degrees. In a large bowl, combine stuffing ingredients, blending well. Stuff lamb and secure with string. Place on rack in oven for ten minutes. Reduce temperature to 350 degrees and slow roast 20 minutes per lb. of meat. Combine raisin sauce ingredients and heat gently, adding a little water to thin, if necessary. During the last five minutes of the meat's cooking time, baste the lamb with the raisin sauce and increase the oven temperature to 400 degrees to glaze. Serve any sauce left over as an accompaniment. Serves 8 to 10.

CHAPTER 3
Alcohol

"If God wanted us high, he would have given us wings." - Arsenio Hall

Mae West once said, "One reason I don't drink is that I want to know when I'm having a good time."

Look to the recipes in the Alzheimer's chapter if you want to improve your memory. One way is not to drink.

These tasty dishes will help alleviate your craving for alcohol, beef up your immune system, especially the liver, which takes the brunt of alcohol's damage, and help you relax your way to sobriety. I've got lentils here for breakfast for the same reason it's in the addictions chapter. Addictions often occur because of an underlying case of depression. Depression can be traced to many causes, one being low blood sugar. Lentils for breakfast is an excellent way to stabilize the blood sugar to get a good start on the day. Look to the chapter on addictions for other excellent lentil recipes.

BREAKFAST

HOT LENTIL CEREAL

1 lb. lentils	1/8 tsp. tarragon vinegar
1/2 cup *pure maple syrup	1/8 tsp. black pepper
juice of 1/2 lime	1/4 cup wheat bread crumbs

Cook lentils well. Allow to cool. Mix with maple syrup, lime juice, vinegar and pepper. Place bread crumbs on top. Place in broiler to brown the top.

*Note: pure maple syrup is very high in nutrients and should not be mistaken for food-free maple-flavored syrup.

LUNCH

FRUITY CARROT SALAD

1 lb. carrots, grated	1/4 tsp. hazelnuts, crushed
1/8 tsp. black pepper	1/2 cup sour cream
1/8 tsp. cayenne pepper	1/4 tsp. honey
juice of 1 lemon	1/2 apple, chopped
1 cup raisins	2 slices pineapple, cut into pieces
Several mint leaves, crumbled	

In small bowl combine all ingredients. Let soak overnight and serve.

DINNER

NUTTY NOODLES

1 cup chopped walnuts	1 tbsp. olive oil
1 clove garlic	2 tbsp. lemon juice
2 tbsp. olive oil	sea salt to taste
2 tbsp. water	

In blender or food processor puree walnuts, garlic and olive oil into a paste (a mortar and pestle made be used instead). Put paste in a small saucepan and heat gently while stirring in remaining ingredients. Add water if sauce becomes too thick. Serve hot over whole wheat or spinach pasta.

OTHER

HOMESTYLE MUSTARD

1 cup low-fat mayonnaise	1 tbsp. lemon juice
1 tsp. tumeric	dash paprika
2 tsp. onion juice	dash garlic
2 tbsp. chopped parsley	dash onion salt

Mix all ingredients in a small bowl. Store covered in refrigerator. Makes about one cup.

CHAPTER 4
Allergies

Food is probably the most common reason for allergy symptoms, although many of us don't know it. Last night I saw a lady that had to leave the restaurant, she was gasping so hard. She had just seen the menu prices!

The foods contained in these recipes have nutrients like vitamin C, to help alleviate allergy symptoms; protein to build up your immune system; and spicy foods that loosen phlegm and help you breathe easier. These foods will help you stay cough-free and dry-eyed even during the heaviest pollen and flu season.

BREAKFAST

PUMPKIN SOUP (hot or cold)

1 two-pound pumpkin, diced
3 oz. chicken or vegetarian stock
1/4 tsp. cayenne pepper
juice of 1 lemon

1 tbsp. no-MSG soy sauce
1 tbsp. chopped fresh dill
1 package cream cheese
1 bunch of cilantro (optional)

Puree pumpkin in a blender or food processor, gradually adding the stock. Pour mixture into a pot and add remaining ingredients. Let simmer for 5 minutes and serve with a dab of cream cheese in the middle or place in the refrigerator and serve cold with cilantro on side of plate as decoration.

TOFU WITH VEGETABLES

1 tsp. vegetable oil
1/4 lb. mushrooms sliced
2 carrots, sliced
1 small onion, sliced
1 cup mung bean sprouts
2 cloves garlic, crushed
1/2 tsp. sea salt

1 cake tofu, cubed
2 tbsp. no-MSG soy sauce
2 tbsp. tahini
1/2 tsp. honey
1 tbsp. tomato paste
1/4 tsp. freshly ground ginger
4 tbsp. freshly chopped parsley

Heat oil in wok or skillet. Add mushrooms, carrots, peas and onions. Stir vigorously about two minutes. Add remaining ingredients. Cover and steam for three minutes. Top with parsley before serving. Serves 4-6.

LUNCH

PEPPER CHICKEN

1 range-fed chicken (health food store)	1/8 tsp. cayenne pepper
1 cup chicken broth	1/8 tsp. lemon pepper
1 small clove garlic; chopped	1/2 tsp. cilantro
1/2 medium onion, chopped	

Season chicken with cayenne pepper and lemon pepper.
Sauce: Add to saucepan: chicken broth, chopped garlic, onion and cilantro. Simmer for ten minutes and serve with brown rice.

WHEEZE-NOT CHICKEN CASSEROLE

1 chicken, cooked and chopped	1/8 tsp. cayenne pepper
2 medium leeks	1/4 tsp. chopped cilantro
1/2 lb. asparagus	1/8 tsp nutmeg
1/2 medium onion, chopped	1/4 tsp. oregano
1/2 cup sour cream	1/4 cup bread crumbs
1/8 tsp. black pepper	2 tsp. parmesan cheese

Dice chicken, leeks, asparagus and onion. Place in buttered baking dish. Add black pepper, cayenne pepper, cilantro, nutmeg, oregano and sour cream. Top with bread crumbs and parmesan cheese. Bake at 350 degrees for 35 minutes or until brown.

DINNER

SPINACH VEGETABLES

1/2 lb. fresh spinach	1/4 yellow onion, diced
1 tbsp. butter	pinch nutmeg
pinch black pepper	1/4 lemon, diced

Lightly steam spinach and set aside. Add butter to hot fry pan and saute onion until just tender. Add spinach and rest of ingredients, saute 3-5 minutes only.

WATERCRESS SANDWICH

> 2 slices nine-grain bread
> 2 tsp. Dijon mustard
> 4 slices cucumber
> 2 slices tomato
> 2 leaves watercress
> 4 tbsp. feta or goat cheese

Spread mustard on slices of bread and add other ingredients.

OTHER

GREEN TOMATO CHUTNEY

> 10-12 medium green tomatoes, cut into 1" chunks
> 1 hot red pepper, seeded and finely chopped
> 1 lemon, seeded and finely chopped
> 1/2 cup fresh ginger root, finely chopped
> 1-1/2 cup raisins
> 2 cloves garlic, chopped
> 2-1/4 cups light brown sugar
> 2 cups cider vinegar
> 1-1/2 tsp. sea salt
> pinch cayenne, if desired

Mix all ingredients and simmer in saucepan 15 minutes or until the tomatoes are tender. Pack into hot, sterilized jars. Seal. Process in boiling water five minutes. Makes about 3-1/2 pints.

CHAPTER 5
Alzheimer's

The advantage of a bad memory is that one enjoys several times the same good things for the first time. - Friedrich Nietzsche (1844-1900)

George Burns jokes that the bright side of Alzheimer's is you are always meeting new people and you can hide your own easter eggs.

Listen to my tape on Alzheimer's to find out how at least one person cured himself using nutrition, supplements, knowledge and, of course, lots of faith in the Almighty.

In the meantime, mend your memory and boost your brain capacity with these delicious meals.

BREAKFAST

EGGPLANT STEAK

1 eggplant	1/8 tsp. nutmeg
1 cup milk	1/8 tsp. black pepper
1 egg yolk	1/8 tsp. cayenne pepper
1/4 tsp. oregano	2 tbsp. virgin olive oil

Do not peel eggplant. Slice into one-quarter-inch thick slices. Dip into mixture of egg yolk, milk, oregano, nutmeg, black pepper and cayenne pepper. Place olive oil in skillet and brown both sides or until eggplant is soft.

PECAN TEA BREAD

1/4 cup whole wheat flour	1 cup date sugar
1/4 cup soy flour	2 eggs, beaten
2 tsp. baking powder	1 cup buttermilk
1/2 tsp. baking soda	2 tbsp. vegetable oil
1/2 tsp. allspice	1 cup chopped pecans

Oil and flour 9" loaf pan. Heat oven to 325 degrees. Sift together flours, baking powder, baking soda and allspice. Stir in sugar. Mix together eggs, buttermilk and oil. Add to dry ingredients, stirring to mix. Mix in pecans. Pour mixture into loaf pan. Bake 40 minutes or until toothpick inserted into center comes out clean. Cool in pan 10 minutes. Remove from pan and cool completely on wire rack.

LUNCH

FRITATA

1 bunch spinach, chopped	3 eggs, beaten
1 bunch Swiss chard, chopped	1 tsp. Italian seasoning
4 zucchini, sliced lengthwise	1/4 cup wheat bread crumbs
1 onion, chopped	1/2 cup grated parmesan cheese
1 clove garlic, chopped	sea salt or kelp
2 tbsp. olive oil	cayenne pepper

Thoroughly wash spinach, chard and zucchini. Drain. Steam spinach and chard lightly. Cool. Saute zucchini and onion in oil five minutes. Cool. (Vegetables can be left in refrigerator overnight.) Combine zucchini mixture with spinach and chard. Mix cheese, bread crumbs and seasoning into eggs. Add salt or kelp, pepper and mix with cooled vegetables. Grease 13" x 9" baking pan. Bake mixture in 300 degree oven for 25 minutes or until firm in the center.

HONEY LAMB

1 5-6 lb. lamb shoulder	1/2 tsp. cumin
1 cup honey	1/2 tsp. Spike
1 clove garlic, finely chopped	4 large lemons
1 cup sesame seeds	2 limes

Cut excess fat from lamb. Puree lemons and limes in food processor or blender. In a large container, marinate lamb in the lemon and lime puree. Refrigerate overnight or up to 48 hours. Broil marinated lamb in 350-400 degree oven 15 to 20 minutes. Combine remaining ingredients; brush on sides of meat and continue to broil, basting every 10 minutes until the meat is tender, about 1-1/4 hours. Serves 4-6.

DINNER

CAESAR SALAD

1/4 cup lemon juice	1 tbsp. anchovy paste
1/4 cup water	1 tbsp. honey
1/4 cup cider vinegar	3 tbsp. grated Romano cheese
1/4-1/2 tsp. vegetable salt	3/4 cup olive oil

1/4 tsp. cayenne

1 clove garlic, pressed

1-1/2 cups whole grain croutons

1 bunch Romaine lettuce

Blend all ingredients except oil in blender or food processor. Blend until smooth. Add oil to mixture gradually while blending at medium speed until mixture thickens. Chill thoroughly.

Prepare salad by gently pulling Romaine lettuce leaves apart. Sprinkle croutons on lettuce and add dressing last. Carefully toss until leaves are thoroughly coated and serve.

BELGIAN ENDIVE AND APPLE SALAD

1 apple

1 endive

juice of 1 lemon

1 tbsp. raspberry vinegar

1/8 tsp. black pepper

2 tbsp. pinenuts

1/4 tsp. chopped cilantro

Slice endive and apple into very thin slices. Add lemon juice, cilantro, black pepper and pinenuts. Sprinkle raspberry vinegar on top and serve.

OTHER

PARSLEY DRESSING

1 bunch parsley, chopped

2 cloves garlic, pressed

1-1/2 cups sesame oil

1-1/2 cups lemon juice

1 tsp. dry mustard

kelp

In blender or food processor blend garlic, oil and mustard. Add parsley, lemon juice and kelp to taste. Mix briefly. Store, covered, in refrigerator. Makes about 3-1/2 cups. Can be used as a cooked cold vegetable marinade, salad dressing or hot vegetable sauce.

CHAPTER 6
Anemia

"The great pleasure in life is doing what people say you cannot do." - Walter Bagehot (1826-1877)

Do you feel physically run down? Do stairs leave you breathless? Is your pep pooped? Your gusto gone? Your enthusiasm exhausted?

It may well be that you're not eating the right foods. These recipes are chock full of natural sourced iron, vitamin B12 and folic acid, all body boosters and anemia enemies. So, eat hearty and run up those steps next time!

BREAKFAST

OATMEAL RAISIN COOKIES

vegetable cooking spray	2 tsp. ground cinnamon
1 cup whole wheat flour	1 cup apple juice concentrate
3/4 cup wheat germ	1/4 cup vegetable oil
1/2 cup rolled oats	2 egg whites or 1 whole egg
1 tbsp. low-sodium baking powder	3/4 cup raisins

Preheat oven to 375 degrees. Coat two cookie sheets with vegetable cooking spray. Set aside. Mix the flour, wheat germ, oats, baking powder and cinnamon in a large mixing bowl. Combine the juice concentrate, oil, egg and raisins in a smaller bowl. Pour the mixture into the dry ingredients and blend well. Drop the batter by teaspoons onto prepared sheet pans, about one inch apart. Flatten each mound. Bake until cookies are slightly brown, being careful not to overcook. They burn easily so check every five minutes.

LUNCH

KATIE'S STUFFED CABBAGE

1 two-pound cabbage	dash pepper
1 lb. lean sausage or ground chuck	1/2 cup raisins
2 eggs, beaten	2 cups chopped tomatoes
1/3 cup soy granules	1/3 cup wheat germ
1/2 cup mild cheese, grated	1 small onion, chopped
1 cup cooked brown rice	1 cup water
1-1/2 tsp. sea salt	

Separate the cabbage leaves gently and drop them into boiling water just until the color brightens. Drain; rinse with cold water. Mix together meat, eggs, soy, cheese, rice, salt and pepper. Place 2-3 tablespoons of the mixture in the center of each cabbage leaf and roll stem over end once, to cover the stuffing. Fold sides toward center, then roll cabbage leaf all the way. Continue until stuffing is gone. Reserve any leftover leaves. Preheat oven to 325 degrees. Oil 2-1/2 to 3 quart casserole dish and line it with leftover leaves. Arrange rolls in dish. Heat water, tomatoes, onion to boiling. Pour over the cabbage. Sprinkle wheat germ and raisins over the top. Cover and bake 1-1/2 hours, adding water as needed. Serves six.

DINNER

BEET SOUFFLE

3 medium beets	1/4 tsp. oregano
1 tbsp. butter	1/8 tsp. rosemary
1 tbsp. honey	1/4 tsp. chopped cilantro
juice of 1/2 lemon	

Slice beets. Place beets in small baking pan with butter, honey, oregano, rosemary and black pepper. Squeeze lemon juice over it and sprinkle cilantro on top. Bake for about 20 minutes at 350 degrees.

CHAPTER 7
Anorexia Nervosa

Contrary to common belief, anorexics do eat. But for them, nutritious meals stand out like a Sumo wrestler at an anorexia clinic.

It's obvious my runner friend has never had to diet. She wanted to increase her speed, so she went on a fast. She lost so much weight, her shorts fell down and she tripped on them, losing the race. True story! Honest!

As enumerated in my best-selling book *Foods That Heal*, many studies find that a zinc deficiency is responsible for this heart-wrenching disorder. The following recipes feature zinc-rich foods.

BREAKFAST

LAMB LOAF

1 lb. ground lamb	1/8 tsp. black pepper
1 egg, beaten	1 tsp. brewer's yeast
1 clove garlic, chopped	1/2 cup wheat bread crumbs
1 medium onion, chopped	1/8 tsp. sage
1/8 tsp. rosemary	

Put lamb in large bowl and add other ingredients in order listed, blending well between. Put mixture in well-oiled large loaf pan and bake at 350 degrees for one hour or until desired doneness. Can be served cold with whole wheat bread and mint jelly as a sandwich. Lots of valuable zinc in this one!

LUNCH

HUNGARIAN CHICKEN

1 three-pound chicken, cut up	1 tbsp. paprika
1 lemon, quartered	1 tsp. sea salt
3 tbsp. vegetable oil	1-1/2 cups yogurt, divided
3 medium onions, chopped	

Rub cut sides of chicken with lemon. Set aside. In large stewing pot, heat oil and saute onions until tender. Add paprika and stir to mix well. Add chicken pieces one at a time, coating well with paprika. Sprinkle in salt then cover and simmer over low heat 30 minutes or until chicken is tender. Remove chicken. Add 1/2 cup yogurt to the pot. Blend thoroughly over low heat. Do not boil. Add remaining yogurt and mix gently. Replace the chicken, coating well with sauce. Serves 4-6.

DINNER

APPLE COMPOTE

1 apple	1/8 tsp. cinnamon
1 tbsp. honey	1 bowl cooked oatmeal

Slice or dice apple and saute in pan containing honey and cinnamon. Serve on top of oatmeal.

CHAPTER 8
Appendicitis

I just read about the latest diet. It's called the moral fiber diet. You can only eat foods that were served at the Last Supper.

Fiber is important to avoid getting appendicitis. Raw foods, especially, are helpful. Bugs Bunny had the right idea.

These recipes use foods high in fiber. Be sure and drink plenty of water too!

BREAKFAST

MAGICAL MILLET SOUP

2 quarts vegetable stock or water
3/4 cups uncooked millet
2 cups sliced zucchini
1 large red onion, diced
2 stalks celery with leaves, chopped
1 cup whole small mushrooms

1 tsp. basil
1/2 tsp. thyme
1 tsp. dried mint
1/2 finely chopped parsley
juice of 1 lemon

Bring stock or water to boil in large pot. Add remaining ingredients. Simmer gently, covered, 30 to 40 minutes.

LUNCH

STUFFED APPLES

1/2 cup yellow split peas
3 cups water
6 medium tart green apples
1/4 cup plus 2 tsp. lemon juice
1 tbsp. olive oil
1 onion, chopped

1/2 lb. ground turkey
1/2 tsp. cinnamon
1/4 tsp. white pepper
1/4 cup chopped parsley
2 tbsp. honey

two cups of water until just tender, about 20 minutes. Add more water if needed. Peas should be tender but dry. Cut about 1/2" off the top of each apple. Set tops aside. Scoop the pulp from each apple, leaving a 1/4" shell. Discard the pulp.

Using some of the 2 tsp. of lemon juice, rub it along the inside of each apple to prevent browning. Heat oil and saute onion until it is tender. Crumble in ground turkey and cook until it is no longer pink. Stir in cooked peas, cinnamon, pepper, parsley and remaining 2 tsp. lemon juice. Use this mixture to stuff each apple.

Place apples in pot large enough to hold them in a single layer. Chop the apple tops and drop in the pot, around the apples. Mix 1 cup water and 1/4 cup lemon juice and pour into cooking pot; NOT over the apples. Bring the contents to a boil over high heat then cover VERY tightly. Lower the heat and simmer over low heat 20 minutes. Uncover the pot and raise heat to keep liquid at a low, steady boil. Cook 10 minutes more, basting apples with liquid often. Remove apples carefully to a warm serving dish. Set aside. Raise the heat again to get the liquid remaining into a full boil. Stir in honey. Cook until liquid is reduced by half. Pour over apples.

DINNER

SPICED PEANUTS

1 lb. raw peanuts with skins	1/2 tsp. paprika
1/4 cup vegetable oil	1/2 tsp. cumin
2 cloves garlic, chopped	sea salt to taste
2 tsp. chili powder	

Spread peanuts in roasting pan. Toast at 300 degrees for 25 minutes, stirring occasionally. Meanwhile, heat oil and cook garlic gently, about 10 minutes, but do not let it brown. Strain oil and mix with spices and salt. Pour spiced oil over peanuts and toss to mix well. Roast spiced peanuts 20 minutes more, stirring occasionally. Drain nuts on absorbent paper. Let cool before storing in airtight containers. Makes 3-1/4 cups.

CHAPTER 9
Poor Appetite

"Is there a principle of nature which states that we never know the quality of what we have until it is gone?" - Richard Hotfstadter

My secretary has a cup which reads, "there are some people who don't have to diet to stay slender. We should search them down and kill them. As lucky as these people may seem, they are suffering.

Appetite loss may be a dieter's fantasy, but for those who can't muster an appreciation for eating food, it can be a nightmare. I picked out some recipes with foods that actually increase your appetite and/or restore nutrients that can cause appetite loss.

Try them and see if you don't start looking forward to mealtimes.

BREAKFAST

ENDIVE COTTAGE CHEESE

2 endives	1/4 cup raisins
1 cup cottage cheese	1/4 tsp. black pepper
3 tsp. chives, chopped	2 tsp. raspberry vinegar
1/4 cup walnuts, chopped	1/8 tsp. paprika

Place endives nicely on a platter in a circle. Place cottage cheese in middle and flatten out. On top of cottage cheese place chives, walnuts, raisins, black pepper and vinegar. Sprinkle with paprika and serve.

LUNCH

CHICKEN CAPPRICCIO

1 four-pound chicken, cut up	1 tsp. basil
1 large onion, chopped	1/2 tsp. oregano
2 cloves garlic, crushed	pinch fennel
2 cups canned tomatoes, chopped	2 tbsp. lemon juice

Combine chicken, onion, garlic, tomatoes, basil, oregano, fennel and lemon juice. Cover and simmer 45 minutes or until done. Serves 4-6.

DINNER

SIMPLE BOILED CHICKEN

1 4-5 lb. chicken	1 tsp. sea salt
1 medium onion, peeled and quartered	1 stalk celery w/ leaves, chopped
2 cloves garlic, chopped	few sprigs parsley
2 carrots, coarsely chopped	pinch of thyme
1 bay leaf	10 cups water

Wash chicken thoroughly, put in very large pot with water and other ingredients. Bring to a boil; cover and simmer over very low heat 1-1/2 hours or until chicken is tender. Serves 4-6.

OTHER

NATURAL FRENCH BAKED CUSTARD

4 cups milk	pinch sea salt
5 eggs, beaten	1 tsp. vanilla
1 cup honey	ground nutmeg

Pour milk in large saucepan; blend in honey with wire whisk. Add eggs, salt and vanilla. Mix thoroughly. Heat mixture until slightly scalded, stirring gently. Pour into 1-1/2 quart glass baking dish or individual custard cups. Sprinkle with ground nutmeg. Place custard containers into 13" x 9" glass baking dish with one inch water in the bottom. Bake at 400 degrees on top shelf of oven one hour, or until custard is firm and slightly brown on top. Serves 4.

CHEESECAKE

crust:	filling:
1 cup whole wheat flour	4 eggs
1/4 cup honey	2 cups cottage cheese
1/3 cup wheat germ	1/2 cup honey
3 tbsp. vegetable oil	1 tsp. lemon juice
1 egg yolk	1 tsp. vanilla
grated rind of 1 lemon	2 egg whites, beaten stiffly

Blend all ingredients together well. Place in a 10" pan and pat to cover sides and bottom evenly. Bake in a 350 degree preheated oven five minutes. In blender or food processor place eggs, cottage cheese, honey, lemon juice and vanilla. Blend mixture a little at a time until smooth. Fold in egg whites. Pour filling into prepared crust and bake 350 degrees 30 minutes or until lightly browned. Let cool.

CHAPTER 10
Arthritis

Save the creaking joints for old houses. When you get aches and pains, it's because your body is trying to tell you something. As you get older, your body becomes quite talkative. However, arthritis need not be!

When George Burns was asked if he had arthritis he said, "I got it when it first came out."

"Allow the disease to heal your life. Begin your journey and become your authentic self. Now." - Bernie Siegal, M.D.

A friend of mine takes cod liver oil every day, and at the ripe old age of 75, has never been afflicted with arthritis. Here are some recipes that will keep your bending places well-lubed and pain-free.

BREAKFAST

FRUIT BALLS

3 tbsp. sesame seeds	4 tbsp. sunflower seeds
1 cup seedless raisins, chopped	2 tbsp. soy granules
1 tbsp. wheat germ	2 tbsp. grated coconut
1 cup unsulfured sun-dried apricots, chopped	

Toast the sesame seeds in a heavy skillet until they begin to "jump." Remove from pan. Mix raisins and apricots together. Add sesame seeds, wheat germ, sunflower seeds, soy granules and one tbsp. of the coconut. Mix well and squeeze into one-inch balls. If it is too sticky, add the remaining coconut. (The stickiness depends on how moist the apricots are.) Store covered and refrigerated.

RASPBERRY COMPOTE

1/2 lb. raspberries	1 tsp. butterscotch flavor
1/2 cup honey	several mint flakes, crumbled

Melt honey in a saucepan. Add remaining ingredients and let simmer for three minutes. Serve over cooked, hot whole grain cereal like millet, oats or barley.

LUNCH

CHICKEN BREAST IN CHERRY SAUCE

4 chicken breasts, skin removed　　5 cloves
juice of 1/2 lemon　　　　　　　　1/8 tsp. black pepper
2 cups cherries (fresh or frozen)　1/8 tsp. nutmeg
1/4 cup honey

Brown chicken breast in buttered pan with black pepper, nutmeg and lemon juice on both sides. In a second saucepan saute cherries in melted honey and cloves. Pour over chicken breast and serve.

RASPBERRY FILET OF SOLE

4 filets of sole　　　　sauce:
1 lb. asparagus　　　　1 cup raspberries
1/2 lemon　　　　　　 1/2 cup honey
　　　　　　　　　　　1/2 tsp. vanilla extract
　　　　　　　　　　　several mint flakes
　　　　　　　　　　　1/2 tsp. black pepper

Poach filets in water to which lemon juice has been added. Steam asparagus. Prepare sauce: saute raspberries with remaining ingredients and simmer for 3 to 5 minutes. Pour sauce over filets. Serve asparagus on the side.

DINNER

BERRY DELIGHT

In a blender or food processor mix:
1/2 cup strawberries
2 small apples, cored
1 small carrot, peeled
1/2 cup grapefruit juice

BERRY BERRY SMOOTHIE

1 cup water　　　　　　　 1/4 lb. blueberries, chopped
3 tbsp. flaked agar-agar　　1/2 cup honey
1/4 lb. strawberries, sliced　1 cup orange juice

Heat water to boiling, add agar-agar and simmer four minutes; set aside. Puree berries in honey in blender or food processor and add 1/2 cup orange juice. To agar-agar mixture add the other half orange juice; mix well. Add mixture to pureed berries and blend thoroughly. Pour into serving bowl and freeze, stirring every half hour until desired thickness.

OTHER

BERRY SAUCE

> 4 cups fresh frozen unsweetened berries, thawed
> 2 tbsp. ground tapioca
> berry juice and water to make 1-1/2 cups liquid
> 2 very ripe bananas

Pour juice off berries into a two-cup measure. Add water to make 1-1/2 cups. Put in blender or food processor. Add bananas and tapioca. Blend briefly. Pour mixture into saucepan, cook over medium heat until thickened. Add berries and heat through. Serve over crepes, pancakes, waffles; in yogurt or over ice cream.

DATE SYRUP

> 1/4 lb. pitted dates
> 1/2 cup water

In saucepan combine dates and water. Simmer over low heat until dates are soft. Mash dates and cook until thick syrup is formed. Refrigerate. Serve on crepes, pancakes or waffles.

CHAPTER 11
Asthma

Norman Cousins has six rules for a good life and one word: quality. On the quality of life he says:

"1) Realize that each human being has a built-in capacity for recuperation and repair.

2) Recognize that the quality of life is all-important.

3) Assume responsibility for the quality of your own life.

4) Nurture the regenerative and restorative forces within you.

5) Utilize laughter to create a mood in which the other positive emotions can be put to work for yourself and those around you.

6) Develop confidence and ability to feel love, hope and faith; and acquire a strong will to live."

Did you know many cases of asthma are actually allergies? Oftentimes, asthma is a severe allergic reaction, rather than an ailment of its own. Look also to the recipes in the allergy chapter if you suspect this is the case.

The recipes here have foods that contain vitamins C and B6, such as yellow onions, shown to help alleviate asthma symptoms. Be sure and use honey that is locally produced for benefit, and once again, drink plenty of water to help flush your system of allergens.

BREAKFAST

BLACK BEANS

2 cups black beans	1/2 cup raspberry vinegar
1/2 cup diced jalapeno pepper	1/2 cup maple syrup*
1/2 yellow onion, diced	1/2 clove garlic, chopped
1 tsp. sea salt	

Simmer black beans for about two hours, covered with water. When done at rest of ingredients. Simmer and serve.

*Note: pure maple syrup is very high in nutrients and should not be mistaken for food-free maple-flavored syrup.

LUNCH

GARLIC CHICKEN

1 chicken, cut up	2 cloves of garlic, chopped
1 medium onion, diced	juice of 1/4 lemon
1/8 tsp. black pepper	1 cup chicken broth
1/2 tsp. Dijon mustard	2 tsp. chopped cilantro
1/2 tsp. capers	

In large fry pan cook onions in hot oil until tender. In small bowl mix pepper, mustard, capers, garlic, and lemon juice. Rub over chicken and add to saucepan. Add chicken and cook until brown. Add chicken broth and let simmer until chicken is tender. Serve sauce over chicken and decorate with cilantro.

DINNER

KARL'S CHICKEN COCONUT SOUP

4 cups chicken stock	1 8-ounce can bamboo shoots
2 cups coconut milk	1 medium yellow onion, sliced
1/4 tsp. nutmeg	4 cloves garlic, pressed
1/2 tsp. black pepper	Tabasco sauce to taste
1/2 tsp. cayenne pepper	1 small Belgian endive, sliced
1/4 lb. small mushrooms	1 tbsp. chopped cilantro

Bring stock and coconut to a simmer and add all ingredients except endive. Let simmer for about 20 minutes and add Tabasco to taste. This soup is great spicy hot. Place sliced endive in individual serving bowls and pour soup on top. Top with chopped cilantro to garnish.

OTHER

HOT AND SWEET YOGURT DIP

1/4 cup apricot preserves
1/4 cup horseradish or to taste
1 cup yogurt
whole grain crackers

Mix preserves and horseradish together. Blend into yogurt. Serve with crackers.

RAGTAG RELISH

2 tomatoes; peeled, seeded and chopped
1 large onion, finely chopped
1 green bell pepper, seeded and finely chopped
1 carrot, pared and finely chopped
1 small cucumber; peeled, seeded and finely chopped
1 tsp. sea salt
1/3 cup honey
2 tsp. cornstarch
1/2 cup cider vinegar
1/2 tsp. pepper

Place vegetables in a saucepan; add salt. Cover with cold water and bring to a boil. Remove from heat and drain. In a large saucepan mix together honey, cornstarch, vinegar and pepper. Bring to a boil. Add the vegetables and simmer 3 to 5 minutes or until vegetables are tender. Chill. Makes about two cups.

BAKED JALAPENOS

several large whole jalapenos   sea salt

Rinse jalapenos. Poke a tiny whole in each, and pour in sea salt. Shake well. Place on baking tray and broil for 5-10 minutes.

CHAPTER 12
Bad Breath

Did you read about the man who got kicked out of a public library because of his offensive breath? He sued and won $250,000. And we used to think bad breath was a liability!

Bad breath may come from the mouth, but it often originates farther down - in the digestive tract. Not enough stomach acid to properly break down food can contribute, as too much refined starch and sugar in the diet can. Check out the recipes in the digestive disorders chapter to help here.

In the meantime, the foods in these recipes, like parsley and mint, can actually clean your breath, as well as your digestion.

BREAKFAST

MILLET SALAD

1 lb. millet, steamed	1/8 tsp. nutmeg
1 medium tomato, sliced	1/8 tsp. black pepper
1/2 tsp. chopped parsley	1 tsp. no-MSG soy sauce
1/2 cup tarragon vinegar	several mint leaves, chopped
1/2 cup chopped green onions	1/8 tsp. black pepper

On serving platter, form millet in a mound in center. Arrange tomato slices around the millet and sprinkle the slices with parsley. In bowl combine rest of ingredients. Mix well, pour over millet and tomatoes, and serve.

LUNCH

PERSIMMON CHICKEN BREAST

2 persimmons, peeled	juice of 1/2 lemon
4 chicken breasts	4 bay leaves, crushed
1/8 tsp. black pepper	mint leaves
1/8 tsp. nutmeg	

Place chicken breast in buttered pan. Add pepper, nutmeg, lemon juice and bay leaves. Brown on both sides. Put persimmons in same pan. Cover. Simmer for 10 minutes. Decorate with mint leaves.

DINNER

CARROTS IN MINT SAUCE

6 carrots, peeled and sliced
2/3 cup salted water
2 tbsp. butter
1 tbsp. honey

1 tsp. cornstarch
1/8 tsp. sea salt
juice and grated rind of 1/2 lemon
1 tbsp. mint leaves, chopped

Cook carrots, covered, in water 4 to 8 minutes until barely tender. Drain, reserving 1/3 cup of the liquid. Sauce: Melt butter in medium saucepan. Combine honey, cornstarch and salt. Stir in butter. Add lemon, mint and reserved liquid. Stir until just thickened. Serving: When ready to serve, add carrots to heated sauce and toss to glaze. Serves 4-6.

CHAPTER 13
Baldness

You know you're in trouble when you stop worrying about your hair having body and worry about your body having hair.

I'm not necessarily talking about male pattern baldness, which is what we usually think of, although these recipes can help there too. Do you know how to avoid falling hair? Step aside!

People lose their hair for a lot of reasons. It helps if you do a bit of sleuthing and find out why. In any case, these recipes are designed to strengthen the hair, and keep it healthy, so what you *do* have will look good!

BREAKFAST

AFRICAN ORANGE SALAD

4 navel oranges	1 cup thinly sliced mushrooms

dressing:
1 tbsp. olive oil	1/2 tsp. lemon juice
2 cloves garlic, pressed	pinch cumin
1/2 tsp. paprika	2 tbsp. chopped parsley
dash cayenne	

Peel and section oranges. Remove all white membrane. Combine orange sections with mushrooms. Chill. Combine dressing ingredients and mix well. Portion orange-mushrooms onto four serving plates and top each with dressing.

LUNCH

BALD MAN'S MEAT LOAF

1/2 lb. ground chuck
1 cup bran flakes
1 cup cottage cheese
2 eggs
2 tbsp. tomato paste
1/2 tsp. thyme

2 tsp. Worcestershire sauce
1/2 tsp. pepper
1 tsp. sea salt
1/2 cup soy granules
1 cup tomato juice

Preheat oven to 350 degrees. In large bowl, mix all ingredients in order listed. Use fork to mix together. Place mixture gently into lightly oiled two-quart baking dish or loaf pan. Smooth top with fork. Bake one hour or until cooked through. Serves 4-6.

DINNER

MUSHROOM SALAD

1/3 cup clam juice
1/3 cup olive oil
2 tbsp. vinegar
1/2 tsp. sea salt
1/4 tsp. tarragon

1/4 lb. mushrooms, sliced
1 red onion, thinly sliced
1-1/2 quart torn salad greens
1 tomato, cut in wedges

In a glass or ceramic bowl, combine the clam juice, oil, vinegar, salt and tarragon. Beat with rotary beater until well-mixed. Gently toss salad greens with dressing, garnish with tomato wedges and serve.

CHAPTER 14
Bedwetting

"There are only two lasting bequests we can hope to give our children. One of these is roots, the other wings." - Hodding Carter

One of the most disheartening experiences of childhood is bedwetting. There can be many causes but studies have shown there is a connection between bedwetting and a magnesium deficiency. See my book *Foods That Heal* for non-nutritional solutions to this problem.

In the meantime, these recipes contain magnesium-rich foods which will help dry up the burden of bedwetting.

BREAKFAST

HIGH-FIBER FIG BREAD

1 cup boiling water	1 cup figs, chopped
1 cup bulgur	1/4 tsp. sea salt

In a large bowl, pour boiling water over bulgur. Soak for one hour and drain. Add figs and salt. Grind mixture in food processor or blender. To serve cold: form into small balls or patties and chill. To serve hot: bake in oiled 8" x 4" loaf pan 30 minutes in 350 degree oven. To serve as a breakfast cereal: form batter in pea-sized balls and bake on cookie sheet until dry. Serve with milk.

LUNCH

BEAN SOUFFLE

1 lb. cooked beans	1/8 tsp. black pepper
1/4 tsp. brewer's yeast	1/2 tbsp. cilantro
1/2 tsp. raspberry vinegar	1/4 cup wheat bread crumbs
1/4 cup honey	2 tsp. sliced almonds

Mix together yeast, honey, raspberry vinegar and black pepper. Add to beans and blend well. Place in buttered casserole dish. Top with cilantro, bread crumbs and sliced almonds. Cook in 350 degree oven 30 minutes or until top is brown.

DINNER

APPLE BROWN BETTY

10 apples	1/2 cup raisins
juice of 1 lemon	1/4 cup melted butter
3 cups coarse bread crumbs	1/2 cup chopped walnuts
1/2 tsp. cinnamon	honey
1/2 cup date sugar	

Slice apples and sprinkle with lemon juice. Place 1/2 cup bread crumbs in bottom of 9" square baking pan. Sprinkle with cinnamon and a little sugar. Dot with raisins. Pour on a little melted butter. Repeat procedure twice more. Place a row of apples over bread crumbs. Sprinkle with a little sugar, cinnamon and chopped walnuts. Add a little butter, dripping it lightly over apples. Cover and cook in 250 degree oven one hour or until apples are tender. Drip honey over top before serving. Serves 6-8.

OTHER

BAKLAVA

4 cups apricot kernels, finely chopped	1 cup melted butter
1 tsp. cinnamon	12 oz. (jar) honey
1 lb. filo or strudel leaves	

Make baklava at least 2-1/2 hours before serving. Grease a 13" x 9" baking dish. In large bowl, combine apricot kernels and cinnamon. Blend well and set aside. In baking dish, place one sheet of filo or strudel leaf, extending it up the sides of the dish. Brush with melted butter. Repeat to make five more layers.

Sprinkle with one cup apricot and cinnamon mixture. Cut remaining filo into 13" x 9" rectangles. Place one sheet of filo in baking dish over apricot mixture. Brush with butter. Repeat to make at least six layers, overlapping small strips of filo to make rectangles, if necessary. Sprinkle one cup apricot/cinnamon mixture evenly over filo. Repeat procedure two more times, placing filo on top of last apricot/cinnamon layer. Trim any filo that extends over top of dish. With sharp knife, cut all layers in a diamond pattern to make 28 servings.

Bake in 300 degree oven 1 hour 25 minutes or until golden brown. While filo is cooking, in one-quart saucepan over medium low heat, heat honey until hot but not boiling. After filo is cooked, remove from oven and let warm. Spoon hot honey evenly over it. Cool on wire rack at least one hour, then cover and leave to cool at room temperature.

CHAPTER 15
Birth Control

Statistics show that if your parents decided not to have children, you probably won't either.

While you're not likely to rely wholeheartedly on food for birth control, believe it or not, there are foods that can actually help! Studies have shown that eating large amounts of peas and barley can induce infertility. I would warn you, however, that it is dangerous to restrict your diet to any one food. Variety may be the spice of life, but it is also essential to good nutrition.

Peas and barley contain lots of fiber and are very good for you, so why not try these recipes?

BREAKFAST

HEARTY BARLEY BREAKFAST

2 cups barley	1/8 tsp. cinnamon
1/4 cup honey	2 tbsp. slivered almonds

Barley can be cooked the night before. Place cooked barley in buttered serving dish. In small saucepan heat honey and cinnamon until hot but not boiling. Pour mixture over barley. Sprinkle with almonds and bake at 400 degrees until top is brown.

LUNCH

KRAUT ROLLS

1 medium cabbage	1/4 tsp. black pepper
1 lb. ground chuck	1/2 small onion, chopped
1 cup cooked barley	1 tsp. chopped parsley
1 tsp. brewer's yeast	

Separate the cabbage leaves gently and drop them into boiling water just until the color brightens. Drain; rinse with cold water. In skillet, heat oil and saute onion until tender. Add beef and brown. Drain any juices and add rest of ingredients. Mix well. Place 2-3 tablespoons of the mixture in the center of each cabbage leaf and roll stem over end once, to cover the stuffing. Fold sides toward center, then roll cabbage leaf all the way. Continue until stuffing is gone. Reserve any leftover leaves. Preheat oven to 325 degrees. Oil 2-1/2 to 3 quart casserole dish and line it with leftover leaves. Arrange rolls in dish. Fasten with toothpicks or twine. Place into a covered pan and bake for about 45 minutes.

DINNER

SPLIT PEA SOUP

24 oz. split peas	1/2 tsp. cayenne pepper
4 quarts beef or vegetarian stock	1/4 tsp. nutmeg
1 clove garlic, pressed	2 leeks, chopped
4 large carrots, sliced	1/4 cup no-MSG soy sauce
1 tsp. black pepper	4 onions, chopped

Cook split peas twice over medium heat, using cold water each time. When cooking for the third time, rinse and add stock and rest of ingredients except the onion. When peas are tender, in approximately one hour, brown onions in a separate pan, and add before serving.

CHAPTER 16
Bladder Infection

"I try to take one day at a time, but sometimes several days attack me at once." - Ashleigh Brilliant

If you have recurrent bladder infections, it is important to know that alternative doctors have successfully used garlic, cranberry and cherry juice to treat it.

BREAKFAST

ICY APPLE SOUP

2 apples, cored and finely chopped	1/2 cup yogurt
1 cup water	cinnamon
2/3 cup cranberry juice	

Make the night before for a refreshing and invigorating breakfast.

Simmer apples in water 10 minutes. Mash, blend or puree. Chill. Lightly blend chilled apple mixture with cranberry juice and yogurt; chill well. Serve with a sprinkle of cinnamon.

LUNCH

CHICKEN LEEK SOUP

1 chicken, cut up	1/4 tsp. black pepper
4 cups chicken stock	1 medium onion, chopped
2 cups water	4 cloves garlic, pressed
4 leek stalks, chopped	Tabasco

Simmer chicken in stock until meat falls off bones. Remove bones and skin. Add rest of ingredients except Tabasco. Add Tabasco to taste before serving.

DINNER

VEGETABLES AND DIP

dip:

2 cloves garlic, chopped

2 green onions, chopped

1 stalk celery with leaves, chopped

1/2 small onion, chopped

1/3 cup chopped parsley

1 cup yogurt

1 tbsp. Worcestershire sauce

Mix all ingredients in blender or food processor until smooth. Serve with carrot sticks, radish wedges, cauliflower florets, celery sticks, broccoli florets and sliced mushrooms.

CHAPTER 17
Body Odor

You know you're in trouble when your deodorant has something your social life doesn't: active ingredients.

A guy lost his job by a nose - his boss' nose that is. What he didn't realize was that if his deodorant didn't work, neither would he.

However, deodorants can't be expected to do it all. If your circle of friends grows ever wider and your distant relatives become even more distant, don't buy a stronger deodorant. Go on a better diet - one that gives you plenty of zinc and magnesium.

BREAKFAST

APPLE BREAD

2 medium apples, finely chopped	2 egg whites
1 tsp. lemon juice	1/3 cup olive oil
1-2/3 cups whole wheat flour	1/3 cup honey
2 tsp. baking powder	1/3 cup skim milk
1 tsp. cinnamon	1/2 tsp. vanilla

Preheat oven to 350 degrees. Spray an 8" x 8" baking pan with non-stick spray. Toss chopped apple with lemon juice. Mix flour, baking powder and cinnamon together in a large bowl. Beat egg whites until stiff, but not dry. Set aside. Mix together oil, honey, milk and vanilla. Stir in apples. Fold apple mixture into flour mixture. When well mixed, fold in egg whites. Smooth mixture into prepared pan. Bake at 350 degrees 35 to 40 minutes or until center tests clean. Cool in pan five minutes. Reverse onto wire rack to cool. Serve with vanilla yogurt.

LUNCH

EASTERN STEW WITH FIGS

3 lbs. boneless lamb, defatted and cubed	2 tsp. dry mustard
2 tbsp. olive oil	2 tsp. dry coriander
1 clove garlic, chopped	2 tsp. cumin

40

1-1/2 cups red wine vinegar
1/2 cup water

1 cup dried figs, halved
sea salt to taste

Heat oil in large stew pot; brown meat. Add garlic to meat just before meat is brown. Add vinegar, water, mustard, spices and figs. Bring to a boil. Cover and simmer 1-1/2 to 2 hours. Salt to taste. Serves 4

DINNER

APPLE HONEY

1/2 cup honey
1/4 cup cilantro, chopped
juice of 1 lemon

1/8 tsp. cinnamon
1/4 tsp. vanilla extract
1 lb. apples, sliced

Place honey into a saucepan and heat thoroughly. Do not boil. Add remaining ingredients and simmer for a few minutes. Remove from heat and add vanilla. Let cool and pour over apple slices. Toss and serve.

CHAPTER 18
Breast Ailments

"Whatever women do, they must do twice as well as men to be thought half as good. Luckily, this is not difficult." - Charlotte Whitton

Among the trials some women face is a disorder called fibrocystic disease. Non-cancerous breast lumps form and sometimes pain and discharge follows. Selenium and vitamin E has shown to be helpful in treating this condition, and the foods contained in these recipes are full of these nutrients.

BREAKFAST

GREAT START BANANA FISH

6 fish filets	3 bananas
3-4 tbsp. olive oil	2 tbsp. pine nuts
juice of 1/2 large lemon	

Preheat broiler. In a shallow baking dish, roll the filets in oil until well coated. Sprinkle with lemon juice. Peel bananas, halve them lengthwise and cut into large pieces. Arrange banana pieces on filets. Sprinkle with oil. Broil until bananas are just beginning to brown, and the fish is almost white. Sprinkle on pine nuts and broil one minute or until they are lightly browned.

LUNCH

RED SNAPPER VERACRUZ

1 tbsp. olive oil	1/4 cup sliced green olives
1 large onion, chopped	1/8 tsp. cinnamon
4 tomatoes, peeled, seeded and chopped	pinch allspice
2 cloves garlic, chopped	1-1/2 lbs. red snapper filet
2 tbsp. lime juice	3 tbsp. wheat germ

Heat oil in skillet, add onion and cook over moderate heat until onion is soft. Add next six ingredients. Cook over low heat, stirring occasionally until mixture thickens. Rinse filets and pat dry. Dip in wheat germ to coat. In a shallow pan coated with oil, arrange filets in one layer. Broil, turning once, until fish is opaque, about three minutes a side, depending on thickness. Place filets on warm platter, top with warm sauce. Serves 6-8.

DINNER

FAVORITE TOMATOES

4 tomatoes   3/4 cup wheat germ
3/4 cup blue cheese, crumbled

Preheat broiler. Remove stem ends from tomatoes. Slice tomatoes thick, about three slices per tomato. Top each slice with one tablespoon blue cheese and one tablespoon wheat germ. Broil until cheese is bubbly. Serves 4-6.

CHAPTER 19
Breastfeeding Problems

"The safest way to double your money is to fold it over once and put it in your pocket." - Frank McKinney Hubbard

Think of your breasts as your child's first savings account, and the milk as the interest that accumulates. The quality of the food you eat determines the amount of interest. To maximize your child's benefit, maximize the quality of the foods you eat.

Certain nutrients are vitally important to your baby's well-being and growth, and are contained in certain foods. To expand your child's bank account, try these recipes.

BREAKFAST

PERSIMMON MOUSSE

2 persimmons	2 tsp. vanilla extract
2 tsp. butter	2 muffins of choice
several mint leaves	1/4 lb. cream cheese

Saute persimmons in butter with mint leaves and vanilla. Place onto a plate with a muffin in the center. Serve cream cheese on the side.

LUNCH

CHICKEN CREAM

1 cup chopped broccoli	4 tbsp. whole wheat flour
1 carrot, peeled and sliced	1 cup milk
1 medium onion, coarsely chopped	3 cups diced cooked chicken
1-1/2 cup chicken stock, divided	sea salt
2 tbsp. butter	pepper
2 tbsp. oil	cooked brown rice
1 cup sliced mushrooms	

Simmer broccoli, carrot and onion in 1/2 cup chicken stock 10 minutes. Set aside.

Heat butter and oil together; stir in mushrooms and cook 2-3 minutes over low heat. Stir in wheat flour. Cook 2-3 minutes. Stir in one cup stock, stirring constantly, then add milk and cook over low heat, stirring 10 minutes or until sauce is thick. Add chicken. Stir. Add drained cooked vegetables. If the sauce is too thick, add some of the vegetable cooking stock. Add salt and pepper to taste and serve over brown rice. Serves 4-6.

DINNER

STUFFED CHERRY TOMATOES

12 large cherry tomatoes   1/4 cup chopped chives
1 cup cottage cheese

Cut stem end from each tomato and scoop out inside. Fill hollow with cottage cheese and sprinkle with chives. Can mix cottage cheese with cream cheese or blue cheese for variety or sprinkle with mint leaves or chopped nuts. Bake for a hot taste treat.

CHAPTER 20
Bruises

A physician friend recently told me about an overweight patient who said, "I'm blue about the black and blue bruises all over my body."

To make sure she was not an abused wife, the doctor asked how she got her bruises."I don't know, she replied. "It seems if I even look at myself bruises appear."

Bruising, which is bleeding under the skin, is most commonly caused by nutritional deficiencies, easily remedied by eating foods like the ones contained in these recipes.

BREAKFAST

BAKED PUMPKIN

4 cups pumpkin, diced	1/4 cup honey
1/8 tsp. cinnamon	several mint leaves
1/8 tsp. black pepper	2 tbsp. cold butter

Steam pumpkin until almost tender. Mix together pumpkin, honey, cinnamon, black pepper and mint leaves. Sprinkle bits of crumbled butter on top and bake for 10 minutes at 350 degrees.

LUNCH

SPINACH PIE

2 cups spinach; chopped, cooked and well drained

1 cup chopped onion	2 tbsp. dillweed, chopped
2 tbsp. olive oil	4 eggs
3 green onions, chopped	4 tbsp. butter
1-1/2 cups feta cheese, crumbled	1/2 cup olive oil
1/2 cup parsley, chopped	2 cups wheat bread crumbs
filo or strudel leaves	

Put spinach into large mixing bowl. Saute onion in 2 tbsp. oil until tender, add to the spinach. Add green onions, feta cheese, parsley and dillweed. Mix well. Beat eggs slightly, add to spinach mixture. Mix well. Preheat oven to 350 degrees. Oil two 8" x 8" pans. Melt butter with 1/2 cup oil.

Cover bottom of pan with filo. Edges may overlap sides. Brush lightly with butter/oil mixture and sprinkle with bread crumbs. Fold over any overlapped edges neatly and add another filo leaf. Brush and sprinkle six layers. Top with half the spinach mixture and brush/sprinkle another six layers, same as the first. Do not brush and sprinkle the last layer. Repeat process for second pan. Bake pies one hour or until slightly brown and puffy. Cut into squares or wedges with sharp knife and serve hot or cold. Serves 12.

DINNER

STUFFED GRAPE LEAVES

1 jar grape leaves (1 lb.)	2 tbsp. chopped fresh dill
1/2 cup olive oil	2 tbsp. chopped fresh parsley
1 onion, chopped	1/4 cup lemon juice
1/2 lb. ground lamb*	3/4 cup raw brown rice
2 cloves garlic, crushed	1 cup hot water
4 green onions, chopped	1/4 cup chopped raisins
	(optional)

Place grape leaves in large colander and rinse with hot water. Set aside.

Heat olive oil in large pot. Add onion and cook until tender. Add lamb and stir until lamb is crumbly. Add garlic, onions, dill, parsley and lemon juice. Mix well. Add rice and stir until rice is clear. Add hot water. Cover and simmer 10 minutes. Remove from heat and stir in raisins, if desired. Cool to the touch.

Line the bottom of a large pot with some of the grape leaves. To stuff leaves, place them shiny side down (veins up). Remove the stems. Place a portion of the filling (approximately 1/2 tsp.) at the stem end of each leaf. Roll toward the center and fold in sides, then finish rolling. Place rolled leaf seam side down in prepared pan. Continue stuffing until all the mixture is used. Cover stuffed leaves with extra leaves. Place a plate over the leaves and press down gently. Add water to a depth of one inch below the top of the stuffed leaves. Cover and simmer about 30 minutes, or until rice is done. Open a leaf to check doneness. Serve warm or cold.

* Soy granules, softened in water and drained, can be used instead of lamb.

CHAPTER 21
Bulimia

"No diet will remove all the fat from your body because the brain is entirely fat. Without a brain you might look good, but all you can do is run for public office." - Covert Bailey

If you know someone who has bulimia, buy him or her a copper bracelet. Seriously! A copper deficiency may contribute toward bulimia, say experts. Copper bracelets may work because the body absorbs some of the mineral through the skin. If you don't believe me, listen to my tape on arthritis. Only small amounts are needed, however.

The foods in these recipes contain copper and other valuable nutrients necessary to physical good health and mental well-being.

BREAKFAST

ENERGY MUFFINS

1-1/2 cups whole wheat flour	2 eggs, lightly beaten
1/3 cup soy flour	2 tbsp. olive oil
1/2 tsp. kelp	4 tbsp. molasses
1/2 cup non-instant powdered milk	1/2 cup raisins
1 tbsp. baking powder	1/4 cup sunflower seeds
1 cup skim milk	

Oil enough muffin tins for 18 muffins. Heat oven to 375 degrees. Mix together flour, kelp, soy flour, powdered milk and baking powder. Stir in milk, eggs, oil and molasses until smooth. Mix in raisins and sunflower seeds. Fill muffin tins about 2/3 full. Bake 20 minutes.

LUNCH

FILET OF SOLE IN HONEY DILL

4 filets of sole	1/2 tsp. dill
1/4 cup honey	1/8 tsp. black pepper
juice of 1/2 lemon	1 medium onion, chopped

Place filets in a buttered baking dish.   Add honey and lemon juice.   Over top sprinkle dill, black pepper and chopped onions. Cook in 350 degree oven until fish separates easily with a fork.

DINNER

PASTA BRAVADO

4 cups spinach pasta	2 mushrooms, finely chopped
6 tbsp. olive oil	5 cups vegetable or meat stock
1 onion, finely chopped	1 bay leaf
1 carrot, finely diced	1 sprig parsley
1 stalk celery, finely chopped	pinch thyme
3 tbsp. whole wheat flour	sea salt
1 tsp. tomato paste	pepper

Over low heat saute onion, carrot and celery in oil until soft. Stir in flour, browning lightly. Add tomato paste, mushrooms and four cups of stock. Add herbs and salt and pepper to taste. Bring to a boil. Cover partly and simmer over low heat 30 minutes. Add 1/2 cup stock, bring to a boil. Reduce heat and simmer five minutes.

Add remaining stock, boil, reduce heat and simmer another five minutes. Strain through cheesecloth-lined sieve, pressing vegetables to extract all juices. Pour strained sauce in clean saucepan. Partly cover and simmer over very low heat until sauce is reduced to about two cups. Serve over cooked pasta.

CHAPTER 22
Burns

It was a chilly, overcast day when the horseman spied the little sparrow lying on its back in the middle of the road. Reining in his mount, he looked down and inquired of the little creature, "Why are you lying upside down like that?" "I heard the sky is going to fall today," replied the bird. The horseman laughed. "And I suppose your spindly little legs can hold up the sky?" "One does what one can," said the little sparrow. - *South Plains Catholic*, Lubbock, Texas

Like the little sparrow, we do what we can to help ourselves. We ask God for assistance and seek true knowledge from alternative physicians, who know the value of nutrition in healing. For example, they've learned that the vitamins A, C and E are valuable in both the prevention and treatment of burns. And since we know which foods contain these important nutrients, I can offer you healing recipes for burns.

BREAKFAST

MASHED SWEET POTATOES

1 lb. sweet potatoes	1 tbsp. butter
1/4 cup half and half	1/4 tsp. black pepper
1 egg yolk	1/8 tsp. cayenne pepper
1/4 tsp. nutmeg	

Cook potatoes very well and peel. Mix all ingredients together and mash well.

LUNCH

DILL CHICKEN EGGPLANT

2 cups cooked chicken	1/8 tsp. pepper
1 medium eggplant, sliced and steamed	1/8 tsp. cayenne pepper
1 cup sour cream	1 onion, chopped

1/4 tsp. dill, divided
1/8 tsp. nutmeg
1/4 tsp. oregano
1/4 tsp. rosemary

1 medium tomato, sliced
6 to 8 mushrooms, sliced
1/2 tsp. parmesan cheese

In small bowl, combine sour cream, half the dill, nutmeg, oregano, rosemary, onion, black pepper, cayenne pepper and onion. Mix well and pour into 1-1/2 quart casserole dish. Add pieces of chicken. Make sure chicken is covered with the mixture. Top with slices of eggplant, then slices of tomato, the rest of the dill, sliced mushrooms and parmesan cheese. Cook in 350 degree oven 30 minutes or until top is brown.

DINNER

FIG AND GRAPE SALAD

1 head red leaf lettuce, shredded
15 fresh figs, quartered

1 cup seedless grapes, halved

mint caper dressing:
3/4 cup olive oil
1/4 cup lemon juice

1 tbsp. capers
1 tbsp. fresh mint, chopped

Combine lettuce, figs and grapes in salad bowl. In small bowl blend olive oil, lemon juice, capers and mint. Pour oil mixture over salad; toss and serve. Serves 4-6.

OTHER

APRICOT SAUCE

2 cups dried apricots
2 cups spring water

2 oranges, sectioned
3/4 cup unsweetened pineapple juice

Soak apricots in water overnight. Put apricots, the water they were soaked in, and oranges in blender or food processor. Blend briefly. Add pineapple juice slowly while blending. Makes about six cups. Use over ham and lamb, waffles, pancakes and yogurt.

CHAPTER 23
Bursitis

When I hurt my ankle, a conventional doctor told me I should slow down. I was getting well before he could cure me. He also said if I don't respond to his treatment, he'll find someone who will.

And you can find a good alternative physician with a little looking. Many of them have a shot in the arm pained by bursitis, an arthritis-like ailment. That's vitamin B-12.

These recipes contain B12 and its host B vitamins to help you attain pain-free movement and keep those joints in peak condition.

BREAKFAST

LIVER STEAKS

4 slices calves' liver	1/4 tsp. paprika
1 tbsp. butter	1 clove garlic, chopped
1/8 tsp. nutmeg	1 onion, thinly sliced
1/4 tsp. cayenne pepper	1 apple, thinly sliced
1/4 tsp. black pepper	

Heat butter in frying pan. Saute garlic until brown. Add liver and cook until crispy. Combine cayenne, black pepper and paprika. Sprinkle on both sides of liver steaks and place in broiler pan. Top with onion and garlic and broil for about 5 minutes.

LUNCH

LAMB SHANKS WITH LENTILS

4 lamb shanks	1/2 tsp. rosemary
2 cloves garlic	dash cayenne
3 tbsp. vegetable or olive oil, divided	2-1/2 cups dried lentils
1 onion, chopped	1/4 cup chopped parsley
2-3/4 cup vegetable or chicken stock	4 green onions, chopped
1/4 cup lemon juice	

Preheat oven to 350 degrees. Slice garlic into slivers; insert slivers into shanks. Brown the shanks in two tablespoons oil, then roast shanks on rack in oven one hour. Place pan beneath rack to catch drippings.

Saute onion in one tablespoon oil until tender. Add stock, lemon juice, rosemary and cayenne. Bring to a boil. Add lentils. Bring to boil. Cover and simmer 1/2 hour. Stir parsley and green onions into cooked lentils along with two tablespoons of lamb drippings. Top with lamb shanks and serve.

DINNER

BERRY SMOOTHIE

2 cups skim milk	1 very ripe banana
2 tbsp. wheat bran	1/3 cup honey
2 cups strawberries	2 tbsp. brewer's yeast
1 cup pitted cherries	

Place ingredients in order given in blender or food processor. Blend until smooth.

CHAPTER 24
Cancer

All the world's a stage. Actually, all the world's a movie and each day is the sequel.

Make your movie healthy. Good nutrition can actually prevent cancer. The evidence has been in for years. I chronicled it in my award-winning book *Nutrition - The Cancer Answer.* Even if you have cancer, you can fight it by eating as well as you can.

Give your body a fighting chance and it will last as long as you do.

BREAKFAST

BROCCOLI CHICKEN SOUP

2 large stalks broccoli	4 carrots, sliced
1 chicken, cut up	1 clove garlic, pressed
4 quarts water or chicken broth	1/2 tsp. black pepper
2 leeks, sliced	1/8 tsp. nutmeg
2 onions, chopped	1 tsp. chopped parsley or cilantro

Skin the chicken, and cook until nearly tender. Add remaining ingredients and simmer until tender. Add chopped cilantro or parsley before serving.

LUNCH

VEGETABLE SPECTACULAR

1 zucchini, sliced	6 cabbage leaves, vein removed
1 yellow summer squash, sliced	5 med. potatoes, peeled and diced
1 cup broccoli florets	3 tbsp. butter, softened
1/2 fresh green peas	black pepper
2 carrots, peeled and cut into sticks	1/4 cup melted butter
1 cup green beans, trimmed	

Steam each vegetable separately. Drain and rinse with cold water. Set aside. Boil potatoes in salt water until thoroughly cooked. Drain. Add salt and pepper to taste and mash thoroughly.

Preheat oven to 350 degrees. With soft butter, thickly coat a two-quart casserole dish. Place broccoli, floret side down, in the center of the dish and surround with a ring of overlapping zucchini slices, then a ring of squash slices, then a row of carrot sticks and green beans; filling the spaces with peas. Top vegetables with a thin layer of mashed potatoes. Sprinkle with salt and pepper. Add a layer of cabbage leaves. Repeat layering process with rest of vegetables, ending with a layer of cabbage topped with mashed potatoes. Add salt and pepper to taste as you go. Pour melted butter over all and bake for 30 minutes. To unmold, run a knife around side of dish and unmold carefully onto serving plate. Serves 4-6.

DINNER

SWEET AND SOUR BEETS WITH GREENS

2 bunches beets with bright green tops	sea salt
2 tbsp. olive oil	dash cumin
2 tbsp. honey	dash rosemary
1/3 cup vinegar	dash nutmeg
1/2 tsp. grated orange rind	fresh parsley
1/4 tsp. cinnamon	yogurt

Cut green tops from beets, reserving one inch of stem to prevent excessive "bleeding." Chop beet greens, then saute in one tablespoon oil for five minutes. Set aside.

Boil whole beets until tender, about 25 minutes. Drain, reserving cooking liquid. Peel and chop beets. In saucepan, combine honey, vinegar, orange rind, remaining oil, cinnamon, salt to taste, cumin, rosemary, nutmeg and 1/4 cup reserved cooking liquid. Simmer over low heat 10 minutes, stirring frequently. Add cooked beets to sauce and warm thoroughly. On serving platter, make a layer of beet greens and spoon beets on top. Garnish with parsley and yogurt. Serve hot or cold. Serves 6-8.

CHAPTER 25
Candida Albicans
(yeast infection)

"I have a simple philosophy. Fill what's empty. Empty what's full. Scratch where it itches." - Alice Roosevelt Longworth

Lately, a host of non-prescription medications have come out to battle this common woman's annoyance: genital yeast infection. But few realize that certain foods work just as well as these expensive salves.

Important in a regimen of yeast warriors are foods that restore the intestine's good guy bacteria, like yogurt, brewer's yeast and torula yeast; and foods that discourage the bad guys, like garlic, horseradish and ginger.

Try these recipes if you want to discourage your invading yeast colonies.

BREAKFAST

HONEY-YOGURT CUSTARD

6 tbsp. honey
2 tsp. orange flower water
1/4 cup wheat germ

4 eggs, lightly beaten
2 cups yogurt

Preheat oven to 325 degrees. Butter a 1-1/2 quart baking dish or six individual custard cups. Add honey, orange flower water and wheat germ to eggs. Beat well. Add yogurt and mix thoroughly. Pour mixture into the prepared baking dish(s). Place custard container(s) in pan containing about one inch very warm water. Bake one hour, or until knife inserted in center comes out clean.

LUNCH

RUSSIAN SHISHKEBAB

3 lbs. lean lamb
4 bell peppers, cut into large pieces
6 red onions, quartered
15 cherry tomatoes
1 bunch cilantro, washed and trimmed

7 cloves garlic, pressed
8 large lemons
2 grapefruit
2 tbsp. seasoned salt
2 tbsp. Spike

Cut lamb into 1-1/2" cubes, place in large bowl. Add onion quarters, cherry tomatoes, cilantro and garlic. Cut grapefruits and lemons in half and squeeze juice into bowl; toss in rinds also. Add seasoned salt and Spike. Gently mix all ingredients together, cover, and allow to marinate in refrigerator 48 hours.

Place lamb, bell peppers, onions and tomatoes on skewers, barbecue over mesquite wood fire 25 to 30 minutes. Serves 8.

DINNER

MARINATED BROCCOLI SALAD

1 bunch broccoli	pinch sea salt
1/2 cup olive oil	pinch cayenne
1/2 cup lemon juice	1 clove garlic, pressed

Break broccoli in small florets and steam in salted water until tender on the outside, crisp on the inside. Meanwhile, beat together remaining ingredients. Pour dressing on drained broccoli. Chill well before serving. Serves 2-4.

OTHER

BERRY TROPICALE

1/2 cup honey	1 egg
1/4 cup lime juice	1 cup yogurt, divided
4 cups whole strawberries, trimmed and washed	

In small saucepan, whisk together honey, lime juice and egg. Cook mixture, stirring, over medium heat until it boils up frothy and thickens - about 10 minutes. Cool. Stir in 1/2 cup yogurt. Mix well. Chill until serving time. Just before serving, fold in remaining yogurt and spoon 1/4 cup sauce over each 1/2 cup of berries. Serves 8.

CHAPTER 26
Carpal Tunnel Syndrome

"The real danger is not that computers will think like men, but that men will think like computers." - Syndey J. Harris

Tingling, painful hands or wrists are the most frequent symptoms of carpal tunnel syndrome, a curious affliction that has become common only since the advent of computers. Many a workers' compensation claim has been paid to secretaries and computer operators who get this disorder after spending hours, days and months pecking away on their computer keyboards. My secretary reversed hers with vitamin B6.

B6, and the foods containing it, has been found to be effective in alleviating these symptoms, and in preventing it, since a deficiency can cause it. Try these recipes if you find yourself rubbing your hands and wrists or wondering why they go to sleep all the time.

BREAKFAST

ASHUREY

1 cup cooked chickpeas	1/4 cup raisins
1/2 cup bulgur	1/4 cup figs, chopped
1/4 cup millet	1/4 cup dates, pitted and chopped
1/4 cup barley	1/4 cup dried apricots, chopped
6 cups water	1/4 cup almonds, chopped
3/4 cup milk	1/4 cup walnuts, chopped
3/4 cup honey	dash rose water
1 tbsp. sea salt	yogurt or whipped cream

Cook chickpeas, bulgur, millet and barley in the water one hour or until barley is tender. Add milk, honey, salt, raisins, figs, dates and apricots. Stir and simmer 30 minutes. Add the almonds, walnuts and rose water. Heat and stir. Serve hot or cold. Garnish with yogurt or whipped cream. Serves 6.

LUNCH

CHATEAUBRIAND STEAK

1 chateaubriand steak
1/4 cup spinach, chopped
1/4 can cream of mushroom soup
1/4 cup jack cheese, grated

1/4 tsp. black pepper
1/4 tsp. cayenne pepper
1/8 tsp. nutmeg
1 clove garlic, chopped

Slice the steak from side to side. Combine spinach, soup and cheese. Spoon over one side of steak, replace other side. Sprinkle pepper, nutmeg, and garlic over steak. Close with toothpicks. Brown in oven approximately 15 minutes at 400 degrees.

DINNER

RUSSIAN BORSCHT

1-1/12 lbs. beef short ribs
2 quarts water
1 onion, quartered
1 carrot, cut into 1-1/2" lengths
1/4 cup cider vinegar
4 medium beets, peeled and diced
1 leek, chopped
1 carrot, diced
4 tomatoes, peeled, seeded and chopped

1 cup chopped cabbage
1/4 tsp. lemon rind
sea salt
pepper
lemon juice from 1 lemon
sour cream or yogurt
minced dill

Place first five ingredients to make stock in large pot. Simmer four hours or until meat is tender. Chill stock thoroughly and skim fat from top. Strain stock and set aside liquid. Remove meat from bones. Discard any fat. Dice meat and return it to the strained stock. Bring stock to a boil. Add next six ingredients. Cook on medium heat or until beets are tender. Add salt, pepper to taste and lemon juice. Serve with dollop of yogurt or sour cream and a sprinkling of dill. Good hot or cold. Serves 4-6.

CHAPTER 27
Cataracts

For thou wilt light my candle; the Lord my God will enlighten my darkness. - Psalm 18:28

Don't let cataracts dim your light. Pray for guidance and nourishment. Vitamin deficiencies have been shown to encourage cataracts; and certain vitamins, like vitamin C, has been shown to slow the formation of cataracts.

These recipes use foods important to the treatment and prevention of cataracts. They taste good too.

BREAKFAST

WISE AND WHEATY BRAN BREAD

3/4 cup cracked wheat cereal	1/3 cup water at 115 degrees
1 tsp. sea salt	1 tbsp. dry yeast
1-1/2 cups boiling water	1/2 cup bran flakes
4 tbsp. vegetable oil	4 cups whole wheat flour
2 tbsp. molasses	cornmeal
3 tbsp. honey	

Mix together cereal, salt, boiling water, oil, molasses and honey. Let stand until cooled to 110 degrees. Mix the 1/3 cup water with the yeast; cover and let stand about five minutes or until the yeast bubbles. Add yeast mixture to cooled cereal mixture. Stir in the bran flakes. Gradually add the wheat flour until the mixture is very thick but doesn't form a ball.

Cover and let rise in warm place 45 minutes. Grease two 9"x5" loaf pans and sprinkle them with cornmeal. Stir dough, and divide it between the two pans. Cover, let rise in a warm place until doubled (45 minutes to one hour). Preheat oven to 450 degrees. Put bread in oven and lower heat to 400 degrees. Bake 50 minute to one hour or until bread sounds hollow when tapped. Cool on a wire rack.

To make rolls, form dough into small balls, place in a greased pan with sides touching, let rise, and bake as for bread. Makes two dozen rolls.

LUNCH

STUFFED PEPPERS

4 green bell peppers	1 tsp. brewer's yeast
1 lb. ground chuck	1/2 tsp. black pepper
1 medium yellow onion, diced	1 can tomato paste
1/4 cup chopped parsley	1 can tomato sauce
1/4 cup cooked brown rice	

In skillet, brown chuck. Drain and cool. In bowl mix crumbled meat, onion, parsley, rice, onion, pepper, tomato sauce and tomato paste. Cut the tops off the peppers. Remove insides. Rinse and drain. Spoon in meat mixture, packing tightly. Put tops back on peppers and place in a buttered pan. Bake for 45 minutes at 350 degrees.

DINNER

WARM SPINACH A LA DONN

4 bunches fresh spinach	1/4 cup chopped tomato
2 green onions, chopped	1/4 cup chopped cucumber
4 strips bacon, chopped	2 hard boiled eggs, chopped
1/4 cup mushrooms, chopped	1/4 cup jack cheese, grated
1/4 cup olives, chopped	1/4 cup raspberry vinegar
1/4 cup green bell pepper, chopped	

Rinse and dry spinach well. Remove stems. Place spinach into a large bowl. In a buttered pan saute onions, bacon, mushrooms, green pepper and olives until mushrooms are tender. Add to spinach. Top with tomato, cucumber, egg, cheese and vinegar. Serves 8.

CHAPTER 28
Cholesterol

"Our duty to God is to make of ourselves the most perfect product of divine incarnation that we can become. This is possible only through the pursuit of worthy ideals." - Edgar White Burrill

Cholesterol is like a shoot-out in an old west movie. It has a black-hatted bad guy, and a white-hatted good guy. LDL cholesterol wears the black hat and is the bad guy. He serves to clog arteries. But for the body's own defenses, it creates the white hatted sheriff, who comes to body's rescue to shoot it out with the bad guy. HDL is the body's good guy cholesterol, and actually helps clear the arteries.

To lower cholesterol, look to foods that contain HDL, like fish, oats and eggplant. To keep your arteries clean and healthy, eat these and the other foods in these recipes.

BREAKFAST

SUPER GRANOLA

7 cups rolled oats	1 tsp. sea salt
1/2 cup soy flour	3/4 cup water
3/4 cup slivered almonds	3/4 cup pitted dates
1 cup millet flour	1 tbsp. vanilla
1 cup shredded coconut	

In large bowl mix oats, flours, almonds, coconut and salt. In blender or food processor puree water, dates and vanilla. Add to dry ingredients and mix thoroughly. Pour mixture in large shallow pan and bake at 250 degrees. Stir every 20 minutes to prevent burning. Bake until golden brown and crisp, about 1-1/2 to 2 hours. Makes about 9 cups.

LUNCH

MAUREEN'S HDL PIZZA

2 large eggplants, sliced	4 green bell peppers, chopped
olive oil	6 jalapeno peppers, sliced
1/4 tsp. tumeric	1 10-oz. pkg. jack cheese slices
1/4 tsp. garlic salt	2 cups spaghetti sauce
8 yellow onions, finely chopped	8-oz. can chopped black olives

Preheat broiler. In 13" x 9" baking dish layer eggplant slices. Brush with olive oil and broil until toasted. Turn eggplant over. Brush with olive oil, sprinkle with tumeric and garlic salt, and broil until toasted. Sprinkle on onion, bell pepper and jalapeno. Broil lightly. Place cheese slices over vegetables. Spoon spaghetti sauce over cheese, top with olive slices. Broil until cheese is melted. Serves 8.

DINNER

SHREDDED BEET SALAD

3 medium beets	1 tsp. no-MSG soy sauce
1/2 cup tarragon vinegar	1/8 tsp. black pepper
1 medium onion, chopped	1/4 tsp. chopped cilantro

Wash and peel raw beets. Grate beets. Mix together tarragon vinegar, onion, no-MSG soy sauce, black pepper and cilantro. Mix well and serve.

CHAPTER 29
Circulation Blockages in Legs

"I hate when my foot falls asleep during the day because I know it's going to be up all night." - Stephen Wright

When pain and immobility keep you from doing what you enjoy most, consider these recipes. They are high in vitamin E, the jet pilot of blood clots.

BREAKFAST

COTTAGE CHEESE CAKE

1-1/2 cups crushed graham crackers	1 tbsp. butter
1/3 cup soft butter	3 tbsp. cornstarch
1/2 cup honey	1 cup buttermilk
3 egg whites	3 egg yolks, slightly beaten
1 cup drained, packed cottage cheese	1 tsp. vanilla

Mix graham cracker crumbs and butter with 1/4 cup honey. Press most of the crumbs into a nine-inch cake or pie pan. Save two tablespoons for the topping. Beat egg whites until stiff.

Beat the cottage cheese with the remaining one tablespoon butter, cornstarch and remaining honey until light. Add buttermilk, egg yolks and vanilla. Beat until smooth. Fold in beaten egg whites. Pour into prepared pan. Sprinkle top with reserved crumbs. Bake at 400 degrees for 25 minutes. Reduce oven temperature to 325 degrees and bake 15 minutes longer, or until knife inserted in the center comes out clean. Chill immediately.

LUNCH

ITALIAN CAPONATA

1 medium eggplant	1/4 cup red wine vinegar
sea salt	1 tsp. honey
2 tbsp. olive oil	pepper
2 cloves garlic, peeled and cracked	8 green olives, pitted and sliced
1 cup finely chopped celery	1 tbsp. capers, rinsed twice
1/2 cup finely chopped onion	
5 med. tomatoes, peeled, seeded and chopped	

Dice eggplant in one-inch pieces. Sprinkle with salt and place in colander for one hour. Pat dry. Heat oil. Saute garlic until lightly brown. Discard garlic. Add celery and onion to oil and saute until onion is soft. Add tomatoes and eggplant. Stir to coat with oil. Add vinegar, honey and a light sprinkle of pepper. Stir.

Cover and allow mixture to cook over medium heat about 20 minutes, or until eggplant is soft, stirring occasionally. Stir in olives and capers. Cover and cook an additional five minutes. Chill and serve cold. Tastes best when it has been chilled several days. It can be frozen for up to six months.

DINNER

MELON COOLER BABY

1 cup diced, ripe cantaloupe	1 tbsp. honey
1 tbsp. lime juice	2 tbsp. yogurt

Puree all ingredients in blender or food processor. Chill. Serves one.

CHAPTER 30
Circulation Problems

He who wears out his britches before his shoes makes too many contacts in the wrong places.

Think of your blood circulation as little messengers, constantly running to and fro throughout your body. If the messengers can't get through to deliver nutrients and oxygen, it means there are blockages - clogged arteries - somewhere along the way. Try these recipes for some neat meals that will keep your blood flowing swift and strong.

Show your body you don't consider it just a one-night stand. Give it regular exercise. It keeps your blood circulating freely, and you'll feel great!

BREAKFAST

BEDOUIN PANCAKES WITH FENNEL

1/4 cup crumbled goat cheese or feta cheese
1/4 cup cottage cheese   sea salt
1/4 tsp. fennel seed   pepper
3 eggs, separated   vegetable oil
1/2 cup whole wheat pastry flour

In small bowl, mash cheeses and fennel seed with a fork. Add three egg yolks, flour, and salt and pepper to taste. Blend. In separate bowl, beat egg whites until stiff. Fold into cheese mixture. Heat oil and griddle. Pour circles of batter and brown both sides. Top with fruit yogurt, fruit, jam or syrup. Try date syrup or berry sauce recipes in arthritis chapter or apricot sauce recipe in the burns chapter.

LUNCH

RATATOUILLI

1 medium onion, chopped	1 tsp. dried basil
1 clove garlic, chopped	1 tbsp. flaked dry parsley
2 tbsp. olive oil	1 tsp. sea salt
2 zucchini, thinly sliced	1 tsp. Worcestershire sauce
1 small eggplant, peeled and cubed	1-1/2 cups cooked brown rice
1 green bell pepper, cut into 1" pieces	1-1/2 cups cooked millet
2 cups stewed tomatoes	

Saute onion and garlic in oil for five minutes. Add zucchini, eggplant and bell pepper and cook 10 minutes more, stirring gently. Add small amount of water if needed. Stir in tomatoes and seasoning. Reduce heat to low, cover pan tightly and cook 15 minutes more. Serve immediately over warm rice and millet.

DINNER

RADICCIO SALAD

1 bunch radiccio   1/8 tsp. rosemary
1 bunch curly leaf lettuce   1/8 tsp. black pepper
1 tbsp. raspberry vinegar   1 tbsp. chopped walnuts
1 tbsp. chopped cilantro

Slice radiccio into small slices and place on lettuce leaves. In small bowl combine rest of ingredients. Mix well. Pour over sliced radiccio.

CHAPTER 31
Colds and Flu

The price of heating has gotten so high, we keep our thermostat turned down real low - which in my house means we stop talking and let our teeth chatter out messages in Morse code.

"The only thing harder to get rid of than a winter cold is a '73 Ford Pinto." - Aileen Foster

Arm yourself against colds and flu viruses by eating healthy and concentrating on foods high in vitamin C. The old chicken soup therapy still holds; as does honey, lemon, garlic and onions. These recipes will keep the warm in and the cold out.

BREAKFAST

*MAMA'S CHICKEN SOUP

1 3-4 lb. chicken	1/2 stalk celery, sliced
2 cloves garlic	1 tsp. kelp
olive oil	1 tsp. black pepper
1 onion	1 carrot, sliced
3 bay leaves	

Clean chicken thoroughly, inside and out. Put chicken in large stew pot. Cover with cold water. Roast garlic in olive oil, add to chicken. Cut onion in half, add to pot. Add bay leaves. Bring to a boil and simmer 10 to 15 minutes. Skim fat from top. Add celery and carrot. Simmer one hour. Remove chicken, strain liquid. Mash celery and carrot and return to broth. Chop or shred chicken, discard skin and bones. Add chicken meat to broth. Refrigerate overnight. Before serving skim fat from top and heat thoroughly. Serves 4.

* Named after Fran Sanchez, owner of Mama's Restaurant in San Francisco

LUNCH

WATERCRESS SALAD

2 bunches fresh watercress	dash cumin
3 tbsp. sesame seeds	dash coriander
1/2 cup chicken or vegetable broth	dash rosemary
1 tbsp. honey	sea salt
1 tbsp. vinegar	

Wash watercress and trim only rough or dirty stems. Separate watercress into four bundles, laying stems together and tying with string. Bring large pot of water to boil and plunge in tied bundles of watercress. Boil 2 minutes. Remove and immediately place under cool running water to refresh. Press out water thoroughly so bundle will retain its shape when string is removed.

Lightly brown sesame seeds in heavy fry pan without oil. Stir constantly to prevent burning until seeds start to pop and jump. Remove from heat. Crush seeds with mortar and pestle or nut grinder. Set aside. Mix together broth, honey, vinegar, cumin, coriander, rosemary and salt to taste. Add sesame seeds and put in food processor or blender. Blend until smooth. Pour honey dressing over watercress bundles. Serves 4.

DINNER

WHOLE BAKED ONIONS

4 large onions
8 bouillon cubes
4 large cabbage leaves

Peel onions and remove enough of the tops to wedge two bouillon cubes in the leaves (two cubes per onion). Wrap each onion in a cabbage leaf and aluminum foil, and pack into a baking dish. Cover and bake one hour at 350 degrees.

CHAPTER 32
Colon

When it comes to the health of your colon, great haste makes poor waste. Food that can be quickly eaten will not be quickly eliminated.

Food takes on added importance when it gets to our body's end zone: the colon. The only thing left by the time it gets to the colon, or lower intestine, is poisonous waste products, fiber and water. Without the fiber, there's nothing to move the poisons through - without the water, nothing moves.

Fiber and water are absolutely essential to good health. It will keep you "regular" as advertisers like to say, and it will keep toxins that contribute to cancer and other life-threatening diseases out of your system. The recipes in this chapter and the constipation chapter that follows are full of necessary roughness so you can win your game of health.

BREAKFAST

FIG CAKE

1 cup butter, softened	1 cup walnuts, finely chopped
1/2 cup honey	1 cup raisins
3 cups fig preserves	1 tbsp. nutmeg
5 egg yolks, beaten	1-1/2 tbsp. cinnamon
3 cups whole wheat pastry flour	5 egg whites, beaten stiff
1 cup plain yogurt	

Cream butter and honey together. Add preserves and egg yolks; beat until smooth. Add flour and yogurt alternately. Add walnuts, raisins and cinnamon. Fold in egg whites. Pour into well-oiled 10" springform cake pan. Bake in 350 degree oven 1-1/2 hours or until knife inserted in center comes clean.

LUNCH

CALIFORNIA TOSTADA

4 corn tortillas	1 cup guacamole
4 tsp. vegetable oil	red chili salsa
1/2 head lettuce, shredded	radishes
2 cups cooked pinto beans	parsley

2 cups bean sprouts   cherry tomatoes

Lightly fry each tortilla in oil. Drain. Top each tortilla with lettuce, pinto beans and sprouts. Garnish with radishes, parsley and cherry tomatoes. Top with guacamole and salsa.

DINNER

LEEKS AND CABBAGE

5 cups water
sea salt
1 cabbage, quartered
6 leeks
1 tbsp. fish sauce
1 tsp. cumin

1 tsp. dill
1 tsp. coriander
1 tsp. olive oil
1 tbsp. vinegar
1/8 tsp. pepper

Plunge cabbage and leeks into boiling water for 10 minutes. Drain and chop coarsely. Mix remaining ingredients and place into oiled baking dish. Bake at 350 degrees for 20 minutes.

OTHER

BEE-NUT BALLS

1-1/4 cup non-instant powdered milk
1 cup unsalted peanut butter
1 cup honey

1 tsp. lemon juice
1/2 cup sunflower seeds
shredded coconut

Mix together milk, peanut butter, honey and lemon juice. Mix in sunflower seeds. Form little balls about 1" and roll in coconut. Store in refrigerator wrapped well. Makes about five dozen.

CHAPTER 33
Constipation

"We are born princes and the civilizing process makes us frogs."
- Eric Berne

Constipation is one of many "civilized" disorders: problems that are a result of our sedate lifestyles and poor diets. But it isn't necessarily a fact of life. A little bran can go a long way, and eight to ten glasses of water can make it go even farther. Try these recipes for tasteful ways to keep things moving along.

BREAKFAST

WHOLE GRAIN CEREAL

1/3 cup whole wheat grain
1/3 cup whole barley grain
1/3 cup whole millet grain
1/4 cup dried, chopped dates

1/4 cup dried fruit
2 cups cold water
skim milk

In saucepan, double boiler or steamer place grains in salted water with dried fruit. Boil five minutes. Cover tightly and turn off heat. Allow to stand without removing cover 20 minutes. Serve with skim milk. Serves 1-2.

LUNCH

GLOW OF HEALTH SALAD

1/2 medium bunch red leaf lettuce, torn
1 cup torn spinach
1 cup broccoli florets
1 cup cauliflower florets
1 stalk celery, sliced
4 stalks watercress, chopped
1/2 cup mung sprouts
1 cup ground or slivered apricot kernels

1/2 cup alfalfa sprouts
1 small red onion, finely chopped
1 medium tomato, chopped
1 large carrot, grated
1 cup cabbage, finely chopped
1 tsp. sesame seeds
1/2 cup lentil sprouts

Combine all ingredients. Mix well. Serve with choice of dressing. Serves four.

DINNER

YOGURT SOUP WITH RAISINS

3/4 cup raisins	1/2 cup chopped green onions
2 cups cold water	1 tsp. sea salt
2 hard boiled eggs, chopped	2 tbsp. chopped parsley
4 cups yogurt	2 tbsp. chopped dill
1 tbsp. vinegar	1 tsp. cumin
3/4 cup skim milk	pinch rosemary
2 cups diced cucumbe	1/2 cup slivered almonds

Soak raisins in cold water five minutes. In large bowl blend eggs, raisins and water, yogurt, vinegar, milk, cucumber, green onions, and salt. Refrigerate at least two hours or heat and serve when thoroughly warmed. Do not boil. Garnish with herbs and almonds.

OTHER

RAISIN CAKE

4 eggs	1/2 tsp. sea salt
1/2 cup honey	2-1/2 cups raisins
1/2 cup whole wheat pastry flour	1 cup slivered almonds

Preheat oven to 350 degrees. In large bowl, beat eggs until fluffy. Gradually beat in honey, flour, salt, almonds and raisins. Pour batter into oiled 9" x 9" baking pan. Bake 30 to 40 minutes until center comes clean.

CHAPTER 34
Cramps

"True fortitude I take to be the quiet possession of a man's self, and an undisturbed doing his duty, whatever evil besets or danger lies in his way." - Locke

CEMP is for cramps. What is CEMP? It's calcium, vitamin E, magnesium and potassium. And there are foods that have all four; perfect for combating any kind of cramp, whether it's menstrual or muscular. CEMP foods are: wheat germ, sunflower seeds, soybeans, almonds, Brazil nuts, pistachios and pecans. These recipes are CEMP-ly creative and delicious!

BREAKFAST

RAISIN NUT BREAD

1 cup soy flour	1 cup raisins
1-1/2 cups whole wheat flour	2 eggs, lightly beaten
3 tsp. baking powder	3/4 cup skim milk
1 tsp. sea salt	1/4 cup honey
1/2 tsp. cinnamon	3 tbsp. vegetable oil
1 cup chopped almonds	

Mix flours, baking powder, salt and cinnamon. Stir in almonds and raisins. Mix eggs with milk, honey and oil. Stir egg mixture into dry ingredients. Pour into oiled loaf pan and let stand 20 minutes. Heat oven 325 degrees and bake one hour and 15 minutes or until done.

LUNCH

HONEY MUSTARD DILLED CHICKEN

1 3-4 lb. chicken	1/8 tsp. cayenne
1 cup chicken stock	1 tsp. honey mustard
juice of 1/2 lemon	1 tsp. Dijon mustard
1/8 tsp. nutmeg	1/4 cup sliced almonds

Saute chicken in chicken stock. Add cayenne, nutmeg and lemon juice. Let brown on both sides. Remove chicken from pan. Add honey-mustard and Dijon mustard to pan ingredients. Simmer five minutes. Pour on chicken and top with almonds.

DINNER

SPINACH DELIGHT

2 bunches spinach, washed and trimmed
4 cloves garlic, chopped
2 tbsp. olive oil
1/4 cup sunflower seeds

Lightly steam spinach. Saute garlic in olive oil. Fold spinach in heated oil and garlic. Toss with sunflower seeds and serve immediately. Serves 6-8.

OTHER

CARROT CAKE

1 cup raisins
2-1/2 cups unbleached flour
5 tbsp. baking powder
1/4 tsp. orange peel, grated
1/4 tsp. lemon peel, grated
1/2 tsp. cinnamon

1-3/4 cup honey
1 cup olive oil
3 egg whites
1 cup spring water
1 cup and 2 tbsp. walnuts, chopped
2 cups grated carrots

Drop raisins in small amount of flour to coat. Sift rest of flour and baking powder. Add orange and lemon peel, and cinnamon. Set aside. In large bowl, beat honey and oil. In small bowl, beat egg whites until frothy. Set aside. Add water to honey and oil. Mix. Add flour mixture and mix well. Add raisins, 1 cup walnuts and grated carrots, one at a time, mixing after each addition. Fold in egg whites. Pour mixture in 9" x 13" glass baking dish. Sprinkle top with 2 tbsp. walnuts. Bake 350 degrees 40-45 minutes.

CHAPTER 35
Cravings

"Temptations are a file which rub off much of the rust of our self-confidence." - Fenelon

When cutting down on sugar means putting only one teaspoon on your frosted flakes in the morning, consider foods to satisfy without adding to your food cravings.

Would you believe lentils for breakfast? Better than blueberry pancakes! Lentils contain complex carbohydrates and fiber. The fiber fills you up, and the carbohydrates keep your blood sugar up. Between the two, you may even feel satisfied through lunch!

BREAKFAST

LENTIL PILAF

1-1/2 cups lentils	1 tsp. nutmeg
3 tbsp. butter	1 clove garlic
1 medium onion, sliced into thin rings	2 tbsp. raisins
1 stick cinnamon, about 2" long	1 tsp. sea salt
1 tsp. cumin	3 cups boiling water
1 tsp. coriander	

Cook lentils according to package directions. Set aside. In heavy two-quart pot, melt butter over medium heat. Add onion, cinnamon, spices and garlic. Stir and saute five minutes or until onion is tender. Add raisins. Stir and saute another five minutes, lightly caramelizing the onion. Add lentils, salt to taste, and 2-3/4 cups water. Bring to a boil, cover, and turn down heat. Simmer 20 to 30 minutes. Pour 1/4 cup boiling water over lentils. Stir quickly and continue to cook on low heat ten minutes. Turn heat off; let pot sit, covered, 15 minutes. Serves 4-6.

LUNCH

LENTIL ONION SOUP

24 oz. lentils	1/2 stalk celery
4 quarts beef or vegetable stock	1 tsp. chopped parsley
1 lb. meat of choice or soup bones	1/2 tsp. chopped cilantro
4 onions, sliced	1 tsp. black pepper
1 clove garlic, pressed	1/2 tsp. cayenne pepper

4 large carrots   1 tsp. oregano

Cook lentils twice over medium heat for ten minutes. Rinse with cold water after each time. Cook a third time, this time for one hour in the stock, adding meat, onion, garlic, carrots and celery. Ten minutes before it's done, add remaining ingredients and simmer for 10 minutes. Add one tablespoon white wine vinegar before serving.

DINNER

ZUCCHINI COINS

4 medium zucchini, sliced
1 tbsp. marjoram
1/2 tbsp. black pepper
2 tbsp. parmesan cheese

Arrange zucchini slices on oiled baking dish. Mix dry ingredients together and sprinkle on top. Broil for five minutes and serve. Serves 4.

OTHER

LOW-CALORIE EGGLESS MAYONNAISE

4 cups water   1/2 tsp. onion powder
1 cup millet flour   1/2 tsp. garlic powder
2 tbsp. honey   1/2 cup vegetable oil
1-1/2 tsp. sea salt   2 tbsp. lemon juice

In blender or food processor blend water and flour. Cook in saucepan until thick and bubbly. Cool. Put two cups of this mixture in blender and add honey, salt, garlic powder and onion powder. Blend well then add vegetable oil until white and shiny, and lemon juice. Store covered in refrigerator. Makes about five cups.

BARBECUE SAUCE

1/2 cup tomato sauce   1/4 tsp. sweet basil
juice of 1 lemon wedge   1 tsp. honey
1 clove garlic, crushed   1 tsp. vinegar
1/4 tsp. rosemary

Mix ingredients well in small saucepan, heat to boiling. Reduce heat to low and simmer five to ten minutes. Use immediately or store in sealed glass jar in refrigerator. Makes about 1/2 cup.

CHAPTER 36
Depression

One of our former presidents, Harry S. Truman, summed it up well: "When your neighbor loses a job, it's a recession. When you lose yours, it's a depression." Of course, that's not the kind of depression I'm talking about. It's the kind that happens within your mind - no matter what the cause.

Depression can be brought on by many things, but can be prevented and treated through good nutrition, certain foods and, always, laughter. Laughter produces chemicals in the body that actually promotes a sense of well-being. It's a tranquilizer without the side effects.

Certain foods contain tryptophan, a natural sedative, and others work to nourish your nerves so things don't *feel* as bad as they seem.

God's word forbids our being depressed. In Isaiah 41:10 He says: Fear thou not, for I *am* with thee. Be not dismayed; for I *am* thy God. I will strengthen thee, I will help thee, I will uphold thee with the right hand of my righteousness.

These recipes are dedicated to Oz's lion, who searched high and low and found courage right in front of him.

BREAKFAST

FRUITY OAT BREAD

1 cup rolled oats	5 cups whole wheat flour
2 cups boiled water	3 cups millet flour
1 large apple	1 cup seedless raisins
1/2 cup chopped, pitted dates	1/2 tsp. caraway seed
2 pkgs. dry yeast	1 tsp. anise seed
1-1/2 tsp. sea salt	

Put oats into a large bowl and pour on boiled water. Let sit until water is absorbed, about 25 minutes. Wash and cut up apple. Put into blender or food processor with dates and enough warm water to make 1-1/2 cups liquid. Blend very well. Pour into a large bowl. Add yeast and stir in. Let sit 10 minutes or until bubbly. Combine salt and flours. When yeast mixture is ready, add raisins, anise seed and caraway seed. Add six cups of flour mixture to yeast mixture two cups at a time, mixing thoroughly between.

Knead dough well. Leave dough in bowl, scatter 1/2 cup flour on top of dough and with heel of hand press into the dough with one firm punch. Then roll dough around, punching and rolling, adding the rest of the flour until dough is no longer sticky. Shape dough in mound in center of bowl. Cover with a damp towel. Let rise two hours until double in bulk. Punch down. Divide and place into two lightly oiled 9" x 5" loaf pans, shaping dough out to ends to cover pans. Cover and let rise again until top is well-rounded, about one hour. Bake 50 to 60 minutes at 350 degrees on rack about four inches from bottom of oven. Or until bread tapped makes a hollow sound.

LENTIL PANCAKES

1 cup cooked lentils	1/4 cup *pure maple syrup
3 eggs	olive oil

Spread lentils on an ungreased pie plate or cookie sheet and roast in 300 degree oven 20 minutes. Lentils should be completely dried out and easy to grind. Grind in nut or coffee grinder, or mortar and pestle until they are powdered into the texture of flour. Set aside.

In large bowl, beat eggs. Add honey or syrup. Mix well. Add ground lentils, blending thoroughly into a batter. Heat oil on griddle and pour small circles of batter, browning on each side. Serve with maple syrup.

*Note: pure maple syrup is very high in nutrients and should not be mistaken for food-free maple-flavored syrup.

LUNCH

SPECTACULAR SUPER SALAD

2 medium potatoes, cooked	1/4 red onion, thinly sliced
1 tbsp. chopped parsley	1/4 bunch watercress, chopped
1 tbsp. chopped green onion	2 cups chopped salad greens
1 tbsp. olive oil	1 large tomato, cut in wedges
1/2 tsp. apple cider vinegar	1/2 avocado, sliced
kelp	1/2 cucumber, cut into spears
vegetable seasoning	1/2 red bell pepper, sliced
3 tbsp. mayonnaise	1/2 bunch radishes, sliced

Slice potatoes, toss with parsley, green onion, oil, vinegar, kelp and vegetable seasoning to taste. Add mayonnaise. Chill until ready to serve. Arrange bed of watercress and greens on serving platter. Mound potato mixture in center and arrange tomato wedges, avocado, cucumber, bell pepper and radishes on greens.

RACK OF LAMB WITH MUSTARD SAUCE

2 two-pound racks of lamb, bones frenched
1/2 cup olive oil   1/2 cup water
sea salt   2/3 cup grape honey or jelly
1/3 cup whole-grain mustard   1 cup fresh grapes

Preheat oven to 400 degrees. Brush racks with olive oil, cover bones with foil.
Place lamb in roasting pan, meaty side up and cook approximately 25 minutes.
Sauce: In saucepan combine mustard, water and grape honey or jelly, adjusting for
taste. Add fresh grapes and heat, stirring frequently until grapes are soft and
mixture is thick. Brush meat with mustard sauce and cook an additional ten
minutes. If you are using a meat thermometer, it should read 145 degrees for rare.
Salt to taste.

DINNER

NOODLES WITH FENNEL

1 lb. bulb fennel   1 12-oz. pkg. spinach noodles
sea salt   grated parmesan cheese

Wash and trim fennel. Cut bulbs in half lengthwise if they are small; quarter them
if large. Put fennel in pot with water to cover, and salt to taste. Bring to a boil;
simmer until fennel is tender. Remove fennel from pot, reserving liquid. Bring
liquid to a boil again and add noodles.   While noodles are cooking, shred fennel
finely. Drain cooked noodles and toss with fennel. Sprinkle generously with
cheese and serve. Serves four.

CREAM OF FRESH TOMATO SOUP

2 cups chopped, ripe tomatoes   2 tbsp. butter
1 medium onion, chopped   2 tbsp. whole wheat flour
1 small clove garlic, pressed   1-1/2 cups milk
1/2 tsp. sea salt   1/2 cup cream
pinch allspice   chopped fresh basil or dill

Mix and mash tomatoes, onion, garlic and salt. Simmer over low heat five minutes
or until onion is soft. Set aside.

In large heavy pot, melt butter. Stir in flour and cook gently over low heat, stirring
every three minutes. Stir in milk; blend well to make a smooth sauce (also called
rue). Strain tomato mixture into sauce; stir remainder through sieve, mixing well.
Heat to boiling. Stir in cream. Garnish and serve. Serves four.

CHAPTER 37
Diabetes
(high blood sugar)

"Life is easier to take than you think. All that is necessary is to accept the impossible, do without the indispensable, and bear the intolerable." - Kathleen Norris

If your blood sugar goes up and down like a yo-yo, start pulling your own strings with a healthful diet. Certain foods control insulin and blood sugar, even to the point of making the hypodermic needle unnecessary. Try the following recipes to control your glucose levels.

BREAKFAST

BUTTERMILK BRAN MUFFINS

1-1/2 cups whole wheat pastry flour	1/3 cup honey
2-1/2 cups bran	1 tbsp. sesame tahini
2 tsp. baking powder	1/2 cup raisins
1 egg	1/2 cup finely chopped walnuts
1-1/2 cups buttermilk	

Preheat oven to 400 degrees. Combine flour, bran and baking powder in large bowl. In separate bowl, beat eggs and add buttermilk, honey and tahini. Mix well. Add wet mixture to dry ingredients and stir until thoroughly blended. Add raisins and walnuts. Texture will be somewhat course and lumpy. Divide mixture between one dozen lightly oiled muffin tins or use paper cups. Bake 20 minutes or until golden brown.

EL RANCHO BREAKFAST LIMAS

2 tbsp. sesame oil	1/4 tsp. cayenne
2 medium white onions, diced	2 tbsp. brewer's yeast
2 stalks celery, finely chopped	2 cups cooked lima beans
1 cup tomato sauce	1-1/2 cups grated cheddar cheese
1 tsp. marjoram	juice of 1/2 lemon
1/4 tsp. celery seed	1 tbsp. no MSG soy sauce
1 tsp. garlic powder	finely chopped parsley

In wok or frying pan, saute onions and celery in oil until golden. Add tomato sauce, spices and yeast. Stir well over low heat. Add limas, one cup cheese and continue to stir. Add lemon juice and soy sauce. Heat thoroughly. Before serving, top each serving with cheese and parsley.

LUNCH

BLACK BEAN SOUP

1 lb. dried black beans	dash cayenne
2 stalks celery w/ leaves, finely chopped	1-1/2 tsp. sea salt
2 large onions, finely chopped	2 tbsp. fresh lime juice
1 sweet red or green bell pepper, finely chopped	

Wash beans thoroughly and soak overnight in water to cover; drain. Add enough water to soaked beans to cover generously. Add celery, onions and peppers. Do not add salt or the beans may not soften. Cook beans until very soft, adding water as needed, about 1-1/2 hours. When beans are cooked add salt and cayenne. Mash beans or puree in blender to make a smooth soup. Stir in lime juice. Serve hot. Serves 4-6.

BECHAMEL NOODLES

1 cup skim milk	1-1/2 tbsp. butter
1 slice onion, about 1/4" thick	1-1/2 tbsp. whole wheat flour
1 bay leaf	sea salt
4 peppercorns	white pepper
pinch ground mace	1 12-oz. pkg. cooked noodles

Heat milk to just below boiling point. Add onion, bay leaf, peppercorns and mace. Heat milk, but do not boil. Strain milk; set aside. Melt butter in small pan; stir in flour. Blend. Stir in half the milk. Over low heat, whisk in remaining milk. Bring to a boil. Stir and simmer two minutes until thick. Season with salt and pepper to taste. Serve over noodles.

DINNER

BARLEY VEGETABLE SOUP

4 carrots, chopped	1 cup barley
3 onions, chopped	1 tsp. sea salt
2 parsnips, chopped	1/2 lb. beet greens
2 stalks celery, chopped	1 cup cooked chickpeas
4 tbsp. olive oil	chopped parsley
2 quarts water or vegetable stock	

In large pot, saute chopped vegetables in oil until lightly cooked. Add water or stock. Stir in barley and add salt. Simmer at least one hour or until barley is tender. During last 15 minutes of cooking, add chickpeas and beet greens. Garnish with parsley. Serves 4-6.

FRUIT BARS

1-1/2 cups whole wheat flour, divided
1/3 cup vegetable oil
3/4 cup & 2 tbsp. honey, divided
2 eggs
1 tsp. vanilla

1 tbsp. brewer's yeast
1 tsp. baking powder
1/2 cup chopped dried pineapple
1/2 cup shredded coconut
1/2 cup chopped walnuts

Heat oven to 350 degrees. Oil 8" square baking pan. Mix together one cup flour, oil and two tablespoons honey. Evenly pat mixture on bottom of pan. Bake ten minutes.

Mix together eggs, 3/4 cup honey and vanilla. Mix 1/2 cup flour with yeast and baking powder. Stir egg mixture into flour mixture until smooth. Stir in pineapple, coconut and walnuts. Spread mixture over warm crust. Bake 15 minutes. Cool on wire rack. Cut into bars.

CHAPTER 38
Low Blood Sugar

"If happiness truly consisted of physical ease and freedom from care, than the happiest individual would not be either a man or woman; it would be, I think, an American cow." - William Lyon Phelps (Cud be!)

Whenever I feel tied up in knots I think of the 23rd Psalm and repeat this phrase: "Thank you Lord for restoring my soul" - and I feel reborn again.

I have learned, in whatsoever state I am, therewith to be content. - Philippians 4:11

Foods such as complex carbohydrates, brewer's yeast and whole grains stabilize the blood sugar, making for a much better outlook on life. To keep people from accusing you of having PMS, try these recipes.

BREAKFAST

BEEHIVE BEAN CURD

1 pkg. (14 oz.) tofu	1/2 tsp. honey
2 tbsp. Chinese oyster sauce	2 tsp. cornstarch or arrowroot
2 tsp. no-MSG soy sauce	4 cups cooked cabbage
1/4 cup vegetable stock	2 tsp. sesame oil

Slice tofu cake into nine pieces. In frying pan combine oyster sauce, soy sauce, stock, honey and cornstarch. Bring to a boil. Add tofu, cover and simmer about 10 minutes. Stir occasionally until tofu absorbs the sauce. Serve on a bed of hot cooked cabbage with sesame oil drizzled on top.

LUNCH

GARDEN BURGERS

1 carrot	2 tbsp. cornmeal
1 small zucchini	2 egg yolks
1 small onion	1 egg
3 tbsp. soy granules	2 egg whites
2 tbsp. wheat germ	1 tbsp. chopped parsley
1/2 tsp. sea salt	2 tbsp. olive oil

Grate the carrot, zucchini and onion together. Mix with soy granules, wheat germ, salt and cornmeal. Beat egg yolks and egg together, and add to vegetable mixture. Beat egg whites stiff but not dry. Add parsley to vegetable mixture and gently fold in egg whites. Oil and heat griddle or heavy skillet. Drop vegetable mixture by teaspoonfuls onto griddle. Cook slowly about four minutes each side. Serve in whole wheat pita bread with choice of accompaniments. Serves 4-6.

DINNER

GRAIN AND BEAN SALAD

1 clove garlic, cut	1/4 cup chopped parsley
1 heaping tbsp. horseradish mustard	1/4 cup chopped coriander leaves
1-2 tbsp. honey	1 bunch green onions, chopped
1 tbsp. fresh dill	2 cucumbers, chopped
1 tbsp. fresh thyme	1 fennel bulb, chopped
1 tbsp. cumin	1 bunch radishes, chopped
1/2 cup olive oil	1/2 cup sliced black olives
1/4 cup wine vinegar	1/2 cup chopped dates
sea salt	3 hard boiled eggs, sliced
1-1/2 cups cooked warm pearl barley	2 tbsp. sesame seeds
1-1/2 cups cooked warm lentils	1 cup crumbled goat cheese

Rub a large salad bowl with garlic and discard. Add freshly-cooked grains. In small bowl combine mustard, honey, dill, thyme, cumin, olive oil, vinegar and salt to taste. Mix well. Pour dressing over grains and blend well. Allow to cool before adding rest of ingredients (except sesame seeds and cheese). Before serving add sesame seeds and cheese. Toss. Serves 6-8.

CHAPTER 39
Diarrhea

"One machine can do the work of fifty ordinary men. No machine can do the work of one extraordinary man." - Elbert Hubbard

Before you reach for the medicine cabinet, consider the fact that diarrhea is the body's way of curing itself. If you eat bad food or have a stomach virus, your body attempts to flush it out. The key to dealing with diarrhea is to drink liquids and eat foods high in potassium, acidophilus and fiber to avoid dehydration, restore the natural balance, and help the body do what it does best.

BREAKFAST

CAROB-HONEY SPONGE CAKE

1 cup whole wheat pastry flour	1/3 cup butter, softened
1/2 cup carob flour	1/2 cup honey
2 tsp. cinnamon	1/3 cup water
1 tsp. nutmeg	2 tsp. grape juice
3 bananas, mashed	6 eggs, separated

Combine flour, carob, nutmeg and cinnamon. Mix well. Beat egg yolks, add butter and honey. Mix well. Add water, bananas and grape juice to egg mixture. Combine the two mixtures and stir thoroughly. In separate bowl, beat egg whites until they form stiff peaks. Fold egg whites gently into batter. Do not overbeat; allow air to be trapped in batter.

Preheat oven to 300 degrees. Pour batter into oiled 9" springform pan. Bake 1-1/4 hours. Or use two 8" x 9" loaf pans and bake one hour five minutes, or until knife inserted in center comes out clean.

LUNCH

BLUE VEGETABLES

2 cloves garlic, chopped	1 cup lowfat yogurt
2 tbsp. minced sweet onion	2-1/2 oz. blue cheese
1/2 tsp. Worcestershire sauce	raw carrot, celery sticks
1/2 tsp. hot pepper sauce	raw broccoli & cauliflower florets

Place everything except cheese and vegetables in blender or food processor. Blend until smooth. Add crumbled cheese to mixture. Blend to desired consistency. For extra lumpy blend only half the cheese and crumble in remaining. Dip vegetables in sauce.

DINNER

PUMPKINSEED PINECONE

1-1/4 cups grated white cheddar cheese (8 oz.)
4 tbsp. yogurt   1 tsp. caraway seeds
1/2 tsp. dry mustard   1/2 cup pumpkin seeds
1/4 tsp. paprika   sesame wafers

Mix and mash everything together except pumpkins seeds. Mix until smooth. Form into a pinecone shape. Chill at least two hours. Garnish chilled mound with pumpkin seeds to resemble a pinecone. Serve with sesame wafers.

CHAPTER 40
Digestive Disorders

Are there days you feel your internally generated gas exceeds the rate of economic inflation in Brazil? Well, then, it's time to get down to causes to achieve better effects.

Fresh, raw food and plenty of water and fiber are the best seeds for your internal garden. To keep yourself "regular" and avoid long-term, chronic conditions, try these recipes.

BREAKFAST

BEAN SALAD

1 lb. dried kidney beans	1/4 tsp. black pepper
1/4 tsp. brewer's yeast	l/4 tsp. cayenne pepper
1 cup white wine vinegar	1/4 tsp. dill
1/4 tsp. oregano	1 tbsp. parsley, chopped
1/4 tsp. nutmeg	1 small onion, diced

Cook beans. Place beans in flat dish. In separate bowl mix all other ingredients. Pour over beans. Marinate overnight and serve.

FIESTA FRUIT SALAD

1 cup mayonnaise	2 cups chopped apple
1/2 cup skim milk	1/2 cup sliced pitted dates
1 tbsp. vanilla	1/2 cup chopped walnuts
2 tbsp. honey	1/2 cup shredded coconut
pinch nutmeg	1/2 cup orange sections
2 cups cubed fresh pineapple	1/2 grapefruit, chopped
3 bananas, sliced	2 tbsp. wheat germ
2 papayas, peeled, seeded and chopped	
2 tbsp. lemon juice	

In small bowl combine mayonnaise, milk, vanilla, honey and nutmeg. Mix well and set aside. Combine all other ingredients in large bowl. Stir until thoroughly mixed. Add mayonnaise mixture and toss until well coated. Serves six.

LUNCH

APPLE SLAW

1 small head cabbage, shredded	1 tbsp. honey
1 carrot, grated	1/2 tsp. sea salt
2 tbsp. chopped celery	dash cayenne
1 tbsp. chopped green bell pepper	1 tbsp. vinegar
1 large apple, cored and chopped	1 tbsp. mayonnaise
1 tbsp. grated onion	

Combine cabbage, carrot, celery, bell pepper, apple and onion in a salad bowl. Mix together honey, sea salt, cayenne, vinegar and mayonnaise. Pour over cabbage mixture and toss well. Let stand at least 20 minutes in refrigerator before serving.

AVOCADO AND SPROUT SALAD

2 cups bean sprouts	2 tbsp. lemon juice
2 cups alfalfa sprouts	2 tbsp. finely chopped onion
1 cup fresh mushrooms, sliced	2 tbsp. chopped pimento
1/2 cup green peas	2 tbsp. mayonnaise
8 dates, pitted and chopped	pinch sea salt
1 large, ripe avocado	

In large bowl mix sprouts, mushrooms, dates and peas. Set aside. In small bowl, mash avocado with fork and add lemon juice, onion, pimento and mayonnaise. Blend until desired consistency. Add salt to taste. Add to sprout mixture and toss. Serves four.

DINNER

PINEAPPLE COMPOTE

1 pineapple	1/2 tsp black pepper
juice of 1 lemon	1/2 cup raisins
1/4 cup choppedcilantro	1/2 cup walnuts
1/2 cup honey	Belgian endives

Dice pineapple and place in pan with melted honey and squeeze the lemon over it. Add the remaining ingredients and saute for 5 minutes. Great on top of a bed of Belgian endives sliced very thin.

ZESTY BRUSSEL SPROUTS

> 1 lb. fresh brussel sprouts
> 2 tbsp. water
> 3 tbsp. lemon juice
> 1/2 tsp. caraway seeds
> 1/4 cup yogurt
> 1 tsp. grated onion

Trim stems from sprouts. Remove all tough and discolored leaves. Steam sprouts in water, lemon juice and caraway seeds 12 minutes or until barely tender. Drain, reserving the liquid. Keep sprouts warm. Add yogurt and onion to reserved liquid. Mix thoroughly. Toss with sprouts. Serve hot.

CHAPTER 41
Ears, ringing
(tinnitus)

If you keep reaching for the phone, only to find the ringing continues, consider the possibility you have tinnitus. Certain nutrient deficiencies have been found to cause it, including B12, manganese and iron.

Look to these recipes for nutrients that can keep your head blessedly quiet.

BREAKFAST

APPLE LIMA STEW

1/2 cup dried lima beans	1/4 tsp. cinnamon
1 onion, chopped	1 cup water
2 tbsp. lemon juice	dash cayenne
1 tbsp. tomato paste	1 tbsp. olive oil
1/2 tsp. sea salt	2 tart apples, cored and diced
1/8 tsp. white pepper	

Soak lima beans in water to cover overnight. Drain. Combine limas, onion, lemon juice, tomato paste, salt, pepper, cinnamon and water. Bring to a boil, cover and simmer over low heat one hour, or until beans are tender. Heat olive oil in skillet. Saute apples five to 10 minutes, until browned evenly. Add to stew five minutes before serving.

LUNCH

MIDDLE-EASTERN BEEF AND BEAN STEW

1 cup dried soybeans	1 bay leaf
3 lbs. stewing beef	3-1/2 cups beef stock
3 medium onions	4 medium tomatoes
2 tbsp. olive oil	3/4 cup raw brown rice
2 tsp. sea salt	1 tbsp. lemon juice
1/4 tsp. cinnamon	

Wash soybeans and cover with cold water. Bring to a boil, remove from heat and let stand one hour. Drain, cover with fresh cold water, bring to a boil and simmer over low heat one hour. Drain. Trim beef, cut into 2" cubes. Cut onions into chunks. Heat oil in large, heavy pot. Brown beef, a few pieces at a time. Remove beef and saute onions until almost clear. Return beef to pot and add beans, salt, cinnamon, bay leaf and one cup of stock. Cover and simmer 1-1/4 hours.

While beef is simmering, drop tomatoes into boiling water for about 15 seconds. The skins should peel off easily. Remove skins and seeds. Chop tomatoes coarsely. Add tomatoes, rice, lemon juice and remaining stock to pot. Cover and simmer 45 minutes or until rice is tender. Serves six.

DINNER

SARDINES IN GRAPE LEAVES

> 1 tsp. lemon juice
> 1 cup olive oil
> 2 tsp. sea salt
> 1/2 cup vinegar
> 1 tbsp. mustard
> 1 cup fresh herbs: dill, mint, thyme, bay leaf, oregano and basil
> 4 lbs. fresh sardines or 2 lbs. fish filets
> 40 grape leaves, fresh-blanched or preserved in brine
> hot mustard

Prepare marinade from lemon juice, olive oil, salt, vinegar, mustard and 1/2 cup fresh herbs. If using filets, cut into two-inch narrow pieces. Marinate the filets or sardines at least one hour. Longer if possible. When ready to assemble, rinse the grape leaves and dry. Place one sardine or filet on the corner, roll up cigar-style, tucking the ends. Use two leaves if one is not enough. The leaves may be secured with string. Grill over hot charcoal coals, ten minutes, taking care not to excessively burn the leaves. Serve with mustard as a dip. Serves 12-20.

Stuffed grape leaves may also be steamed or baked. Steam for 20 minutes. To bake, place in baking pan. Add marinade and bake covered 350 degrees for 30 minutes.

CHAPTER 42
Eczema

"You do what you can for as long as you can, and when you finally can't, you do the next best thing. You back up but you don't give up."
- Chuck Yeager

Ever notice how before and after models are always smiling after? That's because they look better with a smile on. Use these recipes for your eczema, at the same time distracting people with your brilliant smile.

BREAKFAST

AVOCADO VELVET

2 avocados, peeled and sliced
1/8 cup instant mashed potatoes
dissolved in 3/4 cup water

2 green onions, chopped
1/2 tsp. sea salt
1 cup yogurt

Blend avocadoes, potato water, green onions and salt. Fold in yogurt. Serves four.

LUNCH

GOLDEN COLE SLAW

1 cup carrots, grated
1 cup rutabaga, grated
1 cup shredded cabbage

dressing:
2 tbsp. red wine vinegar
1 tbsp. cold water
1 tbsp. white vinegar
1 tbsp. olive oil
1 tbsp. sea salt or kelp
1 clove garlic
1-1/2 tbsp. sorghum

Mix dressing ingredients together thoroughly and toss with combined vegetables.

DINNER

CREAMY CUCUMBER SOUP

2 cucumbers	1 tbsp. chopped parsley
4 green onions	1/2 cup sour cream
1 tbsp. olive oil	1/2 cup yogurt
3 cups vegetable stock	sea salt

Dice one cucumber. Chop green onions and saute in oil until clear. Add cucumber and stir briefly. Add stock and simmer, covered, 10 minutes or until cucumber is very soft. Add parsley and puree in blender or food processor. Seed remaining cucumber and grate it into the puree. Cool to lukewarm. Fold in yogurt and sour cream. Add salt to taste. Chill. Serve cold. Try it on the outside too!

CHAPTER 43
Epstein-Barr Syndrome

There's a new self-help group for people who are too tired to get involved in life. It's called Anonymous Anonymous.

Epstein-Barr is a fancy-named disorder that is actually a virus some say leads to chronic fatigue syndrome and mononucleosis. Sometimes doctors cannot identify it and suggest the patient see a psychiatrist. Alternative physicians know better. They know that vitamin C and exercise is the first step; and after that good nutrition is essential. The foods in these recipes will work to boost your batteries and swell your spirits.

BREAKFAST

STUFFED ZUCCHINI

1/4 cup brown lentils	2 tbsp. olive oil
1 large zucchini	1 medium carrot, grated
1 medium onion, chopped	2 tbsp. wheat germ

Prepare lentils by soaking in water to cover overnight. Place whole zucchini on baking sheet and cook in 300 degree oven until just tender. Meanwhile, rinse lentils and steam until just tender. Saute onion in olive oil until golden and clear. Cut cooked zucchini lengthwise, remove pulp, set aside, and discard seeds. Add grated carrot and lentils to onion, mix well. Add zucchini pulp to mixture, enough to make a moist stuffing. Compress stuffing in zucchini halves and sprinkle with wheat germ. Bake at 300 degrees for 10 minutes.

LUNCH

EGGPLANT TURNIP STEW

1 medium eggplant, diced	1/8 tsp. black pepper
1 medium turnip, diced	1/8 tsp. oregano
1 small onion, chopped	1 cup sour cream
1 clove garlic, pressed	3 oz. jack cheese, grated
2 medium carrots, sliced	2 tsp. grated parmesan cheese
2 tomatoes, chopped	2 tsp. cold butter
1/8 tsp. rosemary	

Combine vegetables in large bowl. In small bowl mix together spices and sour cream. Add to vegetables and mix well. Place in buttered baking dish. Top with jack cheese. Add grated parmesan cheese on top with crumbles of butter. Bake in 350 degree oven 30-40 minutes or until top is brown.

DINNER

CANDIED BEET PRESERVE

8 cups beets, peeled and quartered	1/2 cup water
4 cups honey	2 lemons, thinly sliced
5 tsp. ground ginger	2 cups chopped walnuts

In large pot, cook beets in salted water to cover until almost tender. Drain. Cool and cut beets into julienne strips or cubes. In large saucepan, combine honey, ginger and water. Bring to a boil. Add beets and lemon. Lower heat and simmer one hour or until beets begin to have a transparent look and mixture is extremely thick. Add nuts and cook another five minutes. Serve warm or cold. Makes approximately seven 8-ounce servings. To preserve, pour into sterilized glass jars and keep in a cold dark place.

CHAPTER 44
Improving Your Eye-Q

When a former heavyweight champion began training for a return to the ring, he went on a special diet - a sea food diet. He told the press, "Whenever I see food, I eat."

Well, believe me, there *is* such a thing as a see food diet: better eating for better vision.

The eyes have it. Without them, we're in the dark. Eat foods rich in vitamin C and A to keep your peepers clear and in focus. These recipes are chock full of foods rich in these eye-saving nutrients.

BREAKFAST

FRENCH APRICOT TOAST

1/2 cup apricot nectar	2 egg whites
1-1/2 tsp. cornstarch	1/2 cup skim milk
1/4 tsp. nutmeg or cinnamon	8 very thin slices 7-grain bread
1 large can apricot halves, drained	2-1/2 tbsp. butter
2 eggs	

In large saucepan heat nectar. Stir in cornstarch and nutmeg or cinnamon; cook until thickened. Add apricot halves; heat over low flame to keep warm. Combine eggs, egg whites and milk. Stir to blend. Dip bread in egg mixture, coating on both sides. Saute bread in hot butter until golden. Place one apricot half on each slice and spoon apricot sauce over top.

LUNCH

LAMB STEW

1 lb. lamb, diced	1 tsp. black pepper
4 tomatoes, chopped	1/4 tsp. nutmeg
3 onions, chopped	1/8 tsp. rosemary
4 stalks celery, chopped	1/2 tsp. parsley
4 green bell peppers, chopped	juice of 1 lemon
4 carrots, chopped	2 tbsp. parmesan cheese
1 clove garlic, pressed	several green onions, chopped

In large bowl, combine lamb, vegetables and garlic. In small bowl, combine pepper, nutmeg, rosemary, parsley and lemon juice. Add spices to lamb mixture, blending thoroughly. Place into a buttered baking pan and cook until vegetables have almost dissolved. Add parmesan cheese on top. Serve with green onions sprinkled on top.

DINNER

SESAME CRACKERS AND SPREAD

crackers:

1/3 cup macadamia nuts	1/4 cup rye flour
1/3 cup sesame seeds	1/2 cup wheat germ
2/3 cup water	1/2 tsp. sea salt
1/2 cup millet flour	1/3 cup full fat soy flour, sifted
1/2 cup barley flour	

In blender or food processor, ground macadamia nuts and sesame seeds until slightly pasty. Add water. Blend until smooth. Combine rest of ingredients and paste in a bowl; mix well and knead lightly. If sticky, add more flour. Roll between waxed paper until very thin. Put on a cookie sheet that has been prepared with a thin film of oil. Cut into squares and prick each square with a fork. Bake at 400 degrees 10 minutes or until lightly brown and crisp. Crackers at edges of pan will brown first. Remove them and continue baking the rest. Makes about two dozen.

sesame spread:

2 tbsp. sesame tahini or sesame butter	3 tsp. no-MSG soy sauce
3/4 cup tofu	1 clove garlic, pressed
1 tsp. vegetable salt	1 cup sprouts, chopped if large

Mash everything together except sprouts to make a smooth paste. Mix in sprouts. Serve on sesame crackers topped with tomato slices, cucumber slices, olives or other moist vegetables.

CHAPTER 45
Fatigue

Your strength is gone. You can't lift a finger even to dial the phone. You've been sitting in one place so long you have to clear your throat so the cleaning person doesn't dust you. It's time to try something new: nutrition.

There are many reasons for fatigue, such as low blood sugar, low thyroid function, allergies and anemia to name a few. But getting at the cause can be exhausting. Start with these uplifting recipes to give yourself the energy to look into the whys and wherefors. Then read *Foods That Heal* or get my tapes on fatigue and depression. Call 1-800-445-HEAL.

BREAKFAST

APPLE BAKE

1/3 cup quick-cook rolled oats
1/3 cup wheat germ
1/3 cup hot water
2 tbsp. honey

2 tbsp. molasses
4 apples, cored and sliced
cinnamon

Preheat oven to 350 degrees. Oil an 8" square baking pan. Mix together oats, wheat germ, water, honey and molasses. Arrange sliced apples in baking dish. Top with oat mixture. Sprinkle with cinnamon. Cover dish with waxed paper and bake 30 minutes.

RICE COMPOTE

1 cup cooked brown rice
2 cups water
1 cup chopped dried figs and dates

1/2 cup honey or maple syrup
1/8 tsp. cinnamon
1 tbsp. chopped walnuts

In a bowl mix rice with fruit. Add honey or maple syrup and place into a buttered baking dish. Sprinkle cinnamon on top and decorate with walnuts. Brown in 350 degree preheated oven and serve.

LUNCH

REJUVENATION SALAD

4 large tomatoes, cubed
2 cucumbers, diced
2 stalks celery, diced
1/2 cup finely chopped red onion
1/2 bunch watercress, chopped
1/4 cup chopped parsley

pinch basil
1/2 tsp. dried mint or 1 tsp. fresh
1/4 cup lemon juice
2 tbsp. olive oil
2 tsp. vegetable salt
kelp

Combine vegetables and basil and mint. Toss. Sprinkle with lemon juice, oil, salt and kelp to taste.

LEG OF LAMB WITH BEANS

1 cup dried pinto beans
1/2 cup dried chickpeas
3 cups water
1/2 cup dried lentils
1 five-pound leg of lamb
2 tsp. cumin
2 tsp. dry mustard or 3 tbsp. prepared

1 tsp. parsley, chopped
1 tsp. sea salt
4 cloves garlic, chopped
1/4 cup olive oil
1/4 cup grape juice
2 tbsp. whole wheat flour

Soak beans and chickpeas overnight. Boil together in water 1-1/2 hours, adding lentils after first hour of cooking. While beans are cooking, combine cumin, mustard, parsley, salt, garlic, oil, juice and flour into a paste. Rub paste on lamb. Let stand at least one hour in refrigerator. Preheat oven to 350 degrees. Roast lamb one hour. Turn off oven. Add peas and beans to the roasting pan, stirring in lamb juices. Let stand in warm oven 1/2 hour. Turn on oven to 350 degrees and cook 1/2 hour more. If leg of lamb is over five pounds, add 15 minutes of cooking time for each pound over five.

DINNER

APPLE GAZPACHO

2 tart apples
1 lemon
1 small sweet red bell pepper
1 medium onion

1 clove garlic
2 tbsp. chopped parsley
2 cups tomato juice

Quarter and core apples. Cut off ends of lemon and discard ends. Cut lemon into eighths and discard seeds. Discard stem and seeds from pepper and cut into quarters. Peel onion and cut into 1" chunks. Peel and chop garlic. Puree vegetables, apples and parsley in food processor or blender, in batches, adding tomato juice as needed. Chill overnight to allow flavors to blend. Serve cold.

CAULIFLOWER STEAK

1 medium cauliflower	1/4 tsp. oregano
1 cup milk	1 tbsp. parmesan cheese
1/8 tsp. black pepper	2 tbsp. olive oil
1/8 tsp. nutmeg	1 tsp. chopped parsley
1 egg yolk	

Slice cauliflower into half-inch slices. Dip cauliflower into a mixture of milk, black pepper, nutmeg, egg yolk, oregano, and then in parmesan cheese. Brown in preheated 400 degree oven with olive oil on both sides. Garnish with parsley and oregano.

OTHER

GUACAMOLE

4 medium avocados, mashed	1 clove garlic, pressed
2 small tomatoes, finely diced	juice of 1/2 lemon
2 green onions, finely diced	pinch of cayenne
2 tsp. tamari	

Mix avocados, tomatoes and onions together gently. Fold in seasonings.

CHAPTER 46
Gallbladder

People with gallbladder problems don't need major medical, they need a minor miracle: vitamin E.

Many things have been thought to cause gallstones and other gallbladder problems, including excess fat in the diet. But if the body has enough vitamin E and lecithin, many studies have shown, these problems can be prevented and reversed. Look to the foods in these recipes for your gallbladder-protectors.

BREAKFAST

TOMATO SALAD

4 large tomatoes, sliced	1/8 tsp. nutmeg
1/4 cup lemon juice	2 cloves garlic, chopped
1/4 cup olive oil	4 leaves green lettuce
1 onion, diced	4 tbsp. chopped parsley
1/4 tsp. black pepper	4 tbsp. crushed soybeans

In large bowl, combine lemon juice, olive oil, onion, pepper, nutmeg and garlic. Add tomato slices and marinate overnight. Serve slices of tomato on lettuce leaf topped with one tablespoon parsley and one tablespoon crushed soybeans. Serves four.

LUNCH

GARLIC ANCHOVY BROILED TROUT

4 cloves garlic, chopped	1/3 cup wheat bread crumbs
1/4 cup olive oil, divided	1/2 cup wine vinegar
3 tbsp. anchovy paste or	1/2 tsp. honey
1 two-ounce can anchovies	1/2 cup water
5 small trout filets	fresh coriander leaves

Briefly saute garlic in two tablespoons olive oil. Mash anchovies, whole or paste, into remaining oil. Add garlic, bread crumbs, vinegar and honey. Mix well. Stir in water and simmer on low heat 20 minutes. Prepare fish by slathering sides with warm sauce and broil over high heat until done, about five minutes each side. Or wrap in foil and bake 20 minutes at 350 degrees. Garnish fish with coriander leaves and serve with leftover sauce. Serves five.

DINNER

MIDEAST BABA GHANNOUJ

1 medium eggplant, washed and halved lengthwise
1-1/2 tbsp. tahini | 1/2 tsp. kelp
1/4 cup lemon juice | cayenne
2 cloves garlic, pressed | 1/4 cup chopped parsley

Broil or toast eggplant until skin is blackened. Cool. Peel away skin. Mash pulp until creamy, but not perfectly smooth. Mix together tahini, lemon juice, garlic, kelp and cayenne to taste. Beat into eggplant. Heap into bowl and chill. Serve sprinkled with parsley. Serves four.

OTHER

HOMEMADE MAYONNAISE

1 egg | 7 tsp. lemon juice
1/2 tsp. sea salt | 1-1/4 cup walnut or sesame oil
1/4 tsp. cayenne | 2 tbsp. honey (optional)
4 tsp. apple cider vinegar

Put all ingredients into blender except oil and honey. When mixture is well blended, slowly add oil. Mixture should thicken. If you desire more sweetness, add honey. Makes about 1-1/2 cups.

CHAPTER 47
Intestinal Gas

Do you sometimes feel your internal build up of gas could qualify you as a public utility? You can do something specific and helpful about an intolerable condition that nobody needs to tolerate. And I'm not talking about burping although...

"Everything is worth precisely as much as a belch, the difference being a belch is more satisfying." - Ingmar Bergman

Did you know that in India, to be polite after dining is to belch loudly? No kidding!

Everyone experiences intestinal gas because no one is perfect. We all eat too fast, gulp our food, and binge on food we enjoy.

Gas is our body's way of telling us we need to slow down and consider what's inside. If it happens too often, we need to consider a digestive tune-up, to get things back the way they should be. The foods contained in these recipes will help you settle your stomach and normalize your intestinal tract so you don't have any more of those embarrassing moments.

BREAKFAST

PUMPKIN SALAD

1 two-pound pumpkin	1/2 tsp. chopped cilantro

Cut pumpkin into one to two inch pieces. Steam and cool.

dressing:
1 cup tarragon vinegar	1/4 tsp. black pepper
1 tsp. no-MSG soy sauce	1/2 cup honey

Mix dressing ingredients together and pour over cooked and cooled pumpkin. Decorate with sprinkles of cilantro. Marinate overnight before serving.

LUNCH

CUCUMBER-CHEESE MOUSSE

2 cucumbers, peeled, seeded and grated
3/4 cup lowfat cottage cheese
1 tbsp. chopped chives
1/4 tsp. chopped fresh basil
1/2 cup yogurt
sea salt

pepper
1 bar agar-agar
1-1/3 cups water
1 tbsp. cider vinegar
parsley

Sprinkle cucumber with salt; press between two plates 10 minutes. Drain and rinse with cold water. Oil a ring mold. Mix cucumber with cottage cheese, chives, basil, yogurt, and salt and pepper to taste. Chill. In saucepan, break the agar-agar into water and soak 20 minutes. Cook over low heat 10 minutes. Cool slightly. Stir in vinegar. Stir in 2 tbsp. of cucumber mixture. Stir agar-agar mixture into cucumber mixture. Blend gently but thoroughly. Put mixture into mold and chill. To serve, dip mold briefly into hot water and loosen mousse with knife. Turn onto chilled plate. Garnish with parsley. Serves 4-6.

DINNER

FRUIT SALAD TROPICALE

1 apple
1 orange
1 banana
1/2 cup raisins
1/2 cup diced fresh pineapple

1/2 cup honey
1/4 cup lime juice
1 egg
1 cup yogurt, divided

Combine fruits in medium bowl. Chill. In small saucepan, whisk together honey, lime juice and egg. Cook mixture, stirring, over medium heat until it boils up frothy and thickens - about 10 minutes. Cool. Stir in 1/2 cup yogurt. Mix well. Chill. Just before serving fold in remaining yogurt and toss gently with fruits.

CHAPTER 48
Glaucoma

"The old law about `an eye for an eye' leaves everybody blind."
- Martin Luther King, Jr.

Conventional doctors don't know what causes glaucoma, but alternative physicians have learned what can control it: vitamin C. Try these recipes if you have a family history of glaucoma to increase your odds against it.

BREAKFAST

BAKED OMELET

2 tbsp. olive oil	2 tbsp. yogurt
1 small onion, chopped	kelp
4 eggs, lightly beaten	pepper
1/4 cup grated white sharp cheese	1 tomato, peeled and sliced

Preheat oven to 425 degrees. Heat oil in ovenproof dish or skillet. Saute onions until soft. Mix eggs with cheese, yogurt, and kelp and pepper to taste. Pour mixture over onions. Top with tomato slices. Bake 10-15 minutes or until eggs are set. Serve immediately. Serves 2-4.

LUNCH

VEGETABLE CHOW MEIN

1 cup sliced celery	1 cup broccoli florets
1 cup sliced onion	1/2 cup sliced celery root
1 cup sliced broccoli stalks	2 tsp. vegetable seasoning
1 cup chopped cabbage	1 cup bean sprouts
1 cup sliced mushrooms	2 tbsp. butter

To 1/2 cup boiling water, add vegetables and steam over low heat 15 to 20 minutes. To one cup warm water, add vegetable seasoning; pour over vegetables. Stir in sprouts. Add butter and stir carefully. Serve over brown rice. Serves 6-8.

DINNER

MAPLED APPLESAUCE

>3 large unpeeled apples, chopped
>1/4 cup unsweetened apple juice
>2 tbsp. real maple syrup

Place all ingredients in blender or food processor. Blend at medium speed until smooth.

CHAPTER 49
Gout

"The older you get, the better you get - unless you're a banana."
- Rose, character on *The Golden Girls*

Gout is not a symptom of age. It is caused by a high concentration of uric acid in the blood, which then deposits in joints and crystallizes. Amazingly enough, one food has been found to reverse this. Eminent scientists and doctors have found that cherries and their juice keeps this uric acid from crystallizing. Strawberries, too, have been found to have this property. Try these unique recipes for your gout remedies.

BREAKFAST

DELICIOUS FRUIT-FILLED BUCKWHEAT CREPES

crepes:

1 cup buckwheat flour	1 cup yogurt
1/3 pear or peach juice	2 eggs

filling:

1/2 cup lowfat cottage cheese	1 tbsp. lemon juice
3/4 cup chopped strawberries	dash nutmeg
3/4 cup chopped cherries	yogurt to garnish
2 large bananas, sliced	

In mixing bowl, combine crepe ingredients, blending until smooth. To make crepes, spoon about 3 tablespoons of batter on hot, lightly oiled nonstick crepe or omelet pan. Then swirl batter around quickly to coat pan in thin layer. Cook over medium heat until bubbles appear and it looks dry, about 2 minutes. Then gently turn over and cook other side only about 30 seconds. Remove and cool on clean kitchen towel or on a rack. Repeat to make 7 or 8 crepes.

Blend cottage cheese with fruit and lemon juice in medium bowl. Mix in nutmeg. To fill crepes, place equal amounts of cheese mixture on edge of each crepe. Roll up firmly; place on serving plate seam side down. Garnish with yogurt. Serves four.

LUNCH

CALIFORNIA SUMMER SALAD

1 large cantaloupe	2 cups seedless grapes
or 1/2 medium watermelon, cubed	1 cup mandarin orange segm.
8 bananas, sliced	1 8-ounce can papaya juice
1/2 lb. fresh cherries, pitted and halved	1 quart guava juice
1 pint strawberries, hulled and halved	1 16-oz. carton cottage cheese
4 fresh peaches, pitted and sliced	wheat germ
1 fresh pineapple, peeled, cored and cubed	

Combine all ingredients except cottage cheese and wheat germ in large salad bowl. Chill at least three hours. Serve fruit with scoops of cottage cheese sprinkled with wheat germ. Serves 10-12.

DINNER

BEET SALAD

3 medium beets	1 tsp. no-MSG soy sauce
1 small onion, diced	1/8 tsp. black pepper
1 tbsp. tarragon vinegar	1 tbsp. cilantro

Cook beets in boiling water until tender. Cut in quarters and slice. In large bowl, mix remaining ingredients. Add beets and cover. Refrigerate and allow to marinate overnight.

CHAPTER 50
Gums and Teeth

If you find you're literally putting your money where your mouth is, maybe it's time to consider the dietary connection.

"Be true to your teeth and they won't be false to you." - Soupy Sales

Poor gums and teeth have been connected to a deficiency of over half a dozen nutrients. Even the texture of foods can have a lot to do with gum health. Eating raw, fresh foods not only optimizes your nutritional health, but serves to exercise and maintain healthy gums and teeth.

The following recipes were hand-picked for your eating comfort and pleasure.

BREAKFAST

WALDORF CABBAGE SALAD

1/4 head fresh cabbage, shredded	1 cup mayonnaise
1/2 cup sliced fresh mushrooms	1/8 cup honey
1 small onion, sliced	1/8 cup vinegar
1 tart apple, cored and sliced	1/4 tsp. sea salt
1/8 cup wheat sprouts	1/4 tsp. pepper
1/4 cup alfalfa sprouts	1/4 tsp. kelp
1/4 cup chopped walnuts or cashews	paprika

Toss together all ingredients, except garnish. Top with sprinkle of paprika. Serves 2-4.

LUNCH

SALMON PAPAYA

4 four-ounce salmon filets	1/4 cup honey
1/4 papaya, diced	1 endive, sliced
1/2 tsp. black pepper	1 tbsp. chopped cilantro
1 tsp. dill	raspberry vinegar
juice of 1/2 lemon	mint flakes

On buttered baking pan place salmon filets. Top with pepper, dill and lemon. Brush with honey and top with papaya chunks. Bake in 400 degree oven until fish flakes easily with a fork. On serving plate arrange endive slices then top with cilantro and a splash of raspberry vinegar. Place fish and fruit on top and garnish with mint flakes.

DINNER

MIXED SALAD WITH SOY/YOGURT DRESSING

salad:

1/2 cup watercress	2 green onions, chopped
1 cup torn lettuce	1 green bell pepper, chopped
1 tomato, chopped	2 tbsp. chopped cashews
1 cup coarsely chopped cabbage	1/4 cup grated cheddar cheese
2 carrots, grated	

dressing:

1 cup yogurt	1/4 tsp. rosemary
1/4 cup lowfat soy flour	1/4 tsp. caraway seeds
1/4 cup cider vinegar	

In large bowl, gently toss all salad ingredients together. In small bowl, mix dressing ingredients together. Pour dressing over salad, toss to coat evenly. Serves 2-4.

CHAPTER 51
Hearing Loss

Children today are so accustomed to technology, when mine first found out their grandfather had a hearing aid, they asked if he came with batteries.

What's tragic is that today's technology, most especially electronics that amplify music louder than ears can compensate for, is breeding a generation of the hard-of-hearing. Buy stock in hearing aids now; in 20 years or so, it will sky-rocket. Leaf blowers, jet airplanes and other noisy instruments of modern technology add to the problem.

Fortunately, good nutrition can "immunize" ears against the damage of air pollution. The nutrients contained in these recipes not only serve to discourage hearing loss by guaranteeing against deficiencies; but ensure your hearing organs stay in tip-top shape.

BREAKFAST

BAKED EGGS

> 8 eggs
> vegetable oil
> 2 tbsp. grated white sharp cheddar cheese

Preheat oven to 325 degrees. Oil baking dishes or custard cups that will hold two eggs each. Break two eggs into each dish. Top eggs with cheese. Bake for 10 minutes or until desired doneness. Serves 4.

LUNCH

MANDARIN HERRING

> 4 herring filets
> 2 green onions, chopped
> 1 cup sour cream
> 1/2 cup Mandarin orange sections

> 1/4 tsp. nutmeg
> juice of 1 lemon
> 1 tsp. black pepper

Set aside herring filets. Mix onions, sour cream, nutmeg, lemon juice and pepper together. Place herring on serving platter and top with Mandarin orange sections. Cover with sauce and let soak at least 30 minutes before serving.

DINNER

NUTTY SPROUT SALAD

2 lbs. sunflower sprouts
1/2 lb. pine nuts
2 red bell peppers, chopped
2 bunches seedless red grapes
2 bunches green onions, chopped

2 red apples, cored and chopped
4 stalks celery, chopped
4 carrots, chopped
1/2 cup yogurt

Combine all ingredients then add yogurt to moisten. Serves 6-8.

CHAPTER 52
Heart Problems

"The head never rules the heart, but just becomes its partner in crime." - Mignon McLaughlin

Have a heart for your heart - a change in your lifestyle and diet can make all the difference. There are foods that help the heart in two big ways: by contributing to weight loss and strengthening the Big Pump.

Foods rich in magnesium are the most important to target. A good liquid mineral supplement with magnesium in it works well because it is easily absorbable and gets right where it needs to quickly. However, supplements are no substitute for good food and a healthy lifestyle.

A spiritual base in faith, a daily exercise program, a positive outlook and a diet of raw fruits and vegetables, whole grains, and lean meats and fish help keep my heart strong and efficient, and my health excellent.

These are my favorite heart-starting recipes, try them and you'll see a difference!

BREAKFAST

GREAT BEAN SOUP

1 lb. navy or great northern beans	2 cloves garlic, chopped
1 tbsp. olive oil	3 large tomatoes chopped
3 onions, chopped	2 tbsp. molasses
2 carrots, chopped	sea salt
1 large green bell pepper, chopped	pepper

Soak beans overnight in water to cover. Drain. Add fresh water and cook until soft, about 1-1/2 hours. Do not add salt. Heat olive oil in large kettle. Gently saute onions, carrots, peppers and garlic until onion is just becoming translucent. Add tomatoes, molasses and cooked beans. Stir in enough water to make thick soup. Cook 30 minutes to blend all flavors. Add salt and pepper to taste; cook 10 minutes more. Serve hot.

FRUITCAKE

3 eggs, lightly beaten	1 cup chopped walnuts
1 cup honey	1/2 cup chopped almonds
3/4 cup vegetable oil	3 tbsp. grated orange peél
1 tsp. cinnamon	1/2 cup soy flour
1 tsp. allspice	1 cup non-instant powdered milk
1 cup chopped pitted dates	1 cup wheat germ
1 cup chopped pitted prunes	3 cups whole wheat flour
1 cup chopped dried apricots	1/4 tsp. sea salt
2 cups raisins	1/4 cup boiling water
3 slices dried pineapple, chopped	1-1/2 tsp. baking soda

Line five small 7" loaf pans with parchment. Heat oven to 350 degrees. Combine eggs, honey and oil. Beat two minutes or until thick and creamy. Beat in cinnamon and allspice. Mix in fruits, nuts and orange peel. Add soy flour, milk powder and wheat germ, one at a time, beating well after each addition. Sift wheat flour together with salt and stir into batter. Add baking soda to boiling water and stir into batter. Bake 30-35 minutes or until lightly brown and firm. Cool slightly before removing from pans. Cool and wrap to store. Keeps up to three months in refrigerator.

LUNCH

GOLDEN FRUIT SALAD

3 tbsp. honey	3 bananas, sliced
1-1/2 tbsp. cornstarch	2 papayas, seeded and chopped
1/2 cup pineapple juice	2 cups chopped apple
1 tbsp. grated orange peel	1/2 cup sliced pitted dates
2 tbsp. lemon juice	1/2 cup chopped walnuts
2 tbsp. orange juice	1/2 cup orange sections
2 cups cubed fresh pineapple	2 tbsp. wheat germ

Mix honey and cornstarch in saucepan. Stir in pineapple juice. Cook until thick, stirring constantly. Blend in orange peel, lemon juice and orange juice. Cool. In large bowl, combine remaining ingredients. Gently fold in sauce and serve.

HERRING SALAD

4 herring, sliced	1 pkg. cream cheese
2 medium beets, sliced	1/4 tsp. dill
1 medium onion, sliced	1/4 tsp. pepper
1 large potato, sliced and cooked	

Combine all ingredients in large bowl except herring. Mix well and add herring. Marinate overnight. Can be served warm or cold.

DINNER

TOMATO ICE

1-1/4 cups tomato sauce	2 tbsp. lemon juice
1 clove garlic, crushed	3 slices fresh ginger
1 onion, sliced	1 tsp. Worcestershire sauce
1 stalk celery with leaf, sliced	1/2 tsp. cayenne
1 carrot, sliced	1 egg white
1 tbsp. no-MSG soy sauce	1 thinly sliced cucumber
1 tsp. fresh lemon rind	or 4 avocado halves

Heat together tomato sauce, garlic, onion, celery, carrot, soy sauce, lemon rind, juice and ginger. Bring to a boil; cover and simmer 10 minutes. Press mixture through a fine sieve. Cool. Stir in Worcestershire sauce and cayenne. Place mixture in an ice cube tray or metal pan. Freeze, covered, until almost firm. Scoop into a bowl and beat with wire whisk to break up ice crystals. Beat egg white into stiff peaks and stir into tomato mixture. Freeze until almost firm and whisk as before. Return to freezer for about an hour before serving. To serve, layer in parfait glasses with thinly sliced cucumber or scoop in chilled avocado half. Serves four.

LIQUID SALAD IN A GLASS

3/4 cup finely chopped onion	1 tbsp. olive oil
3/4 tsp. pressed garlic	1/2 cup lemon juice
1-1/2 cups chopped green bell pepper	1 cup water
3-1/2 cups diced tomato	1 tbsp. kelp
1 tbsp. paprika	1/2 cup thinly sliced cucumber

Blend all ingredients together except cucumber in blender or food processor. Chill two to three hours. Blend in cucumber just before serving. Serves two.

CHAPTER 53
Hemorrhoids

Whatever the mind can conceive and believe, the body can achieve. At the risk of repeating myself: fiber, fiber, fiber, water, water, water.

Many digestive disorders arise from a lack of fiber and water. Hemorrhoids are no exception. The key is in finding delicious foods that offer lots of fiber. That's where this book comes in. Try the recipes here, as well as the ones in the appendicitis, colon and constipation chapters to give your hemorrhoids a chance to heal.

BREAKFAST

RAISIN, MILLET AND APRICOT BAKE

1 cup millet	1/2 tsp. ground ginger
2 cups water	1/4 tsp. cinnamon
1/2 cup dried apricots	1/4 tsp. nutmeg
1/2 cup light raisins	butter
1/2 cup dark raisins	yogurt
1/4 cup honey	

Cook millet in one cup water for 30 minutes. Drain. In large bowl, cover apricots and raisins with one cup water. Let stand 10 minutes. Add partially cooked millet, honey and spices. Blend well. Pour mixture into an oiled, 8" x 8" baking pan and dot with butter. Bake in 350 degree oven 40 minutes. Serve warm or cold.

LUNCH

VEGETABLE STROGANOFF

2 tbsp. vegetable oil	1 tsp. Dijon mustard
1 tbsp. butter	2 cups cooked broccoli,
1 large onion, thinly sliced	carrots and cauliflower
3 tbsp. whole wheat flour	1/2 cup cooked mushrooms
1 cup vegetable or chicken stock	1 cup yogurt

Heat vegetable oil and butter together until butter melts. Saute onion in mixture until just clear. Add flour, stir to mix well. Add stock gradually while stirring. Add mustard. Mix well and simmer over low heat; stirring until sauce thickens, about five minutes. Add hot vegetables and mushrooms. Remove from heat and stir in yogurt. Serve over hot cooked noodles. Serves four.

DINNER

CABBAGE SALAD

1 cabbage, thinly sliced	1/2 cup walnuts
2 cups sour cream	1 tbsp. no-MSG soy sauce
1 tsp. black pepper	1/2 apple, thinly sliced
1/4 tsp. cayenne	juice of 1 lemon
1/2 cup raisins	1/3 cup crushed pineapple
1/2 cup honey	

Combine all ingredients but cabbage. Add cabbage and mix well. Refrigerate for one hour and serve.

CHAPTER 54
Herpes

At my high school reunion I overhead two men talking about one of our former classmates. One said to the other, "Is she unattached?" The other replied, "No, just put together funny."

Just because you have genital herpes doesn't mean you can't enjoy a satisfying sex life with your wife or husband. Don't underestimate yourself. What if Michelangelo had said "I don't do ceilings," or Charles Dickens had called his book *Modest Expectations*?

The recipes in this chapter contain nutrients that will help you control your stress levels, which contribute to herpes outbreaks; and foods that condition your skin so the outbreaks won't be so severe.

BREAKFAST

ITALIAN PAN BAGNA

1 large loaf whole wheat french bread	1 tsp. capers
3 tomatoes, peeled, seeded and chopped	1 tbsp. grated parmesan cheese
4 green onions, chopped	2 tbsp. olive oil
1/2 cup chopped, pitted black olives	2 green bell peppers, chopped
1/2 cup chopped, pitted green olives	1 sweet onion, finely chopped
2 tbsp. chopped parsley	lemon juice

Cut the ends from the bread. Using a long spoon, hollow the loaf, reserving crumbs. Mix bread crumbs with the tomatoes, green onions, olives, parsley, capers, cheese, oil, peppers and onion. Mix well. Moisten and season to taste with lemon juice. Stuff mixture into hollow loaf. Wrap the loaf tightly and chill well. To serve, unwrap loaf and cut into 1-1/2" slices.

LUNCH

OVEN-BAKED NO-FAT CHICKEN

1 3-4 lb. chicken, cut up	2 tbsp. dillweed
juice of 1 lemon	1 tsp. paprika

2 egg whites
1/2 cup oat bran
1/4 cup corn meal
1/4 cup wheat germ

2 tsp. garlic powder
1 tsp. dry mustard
1 tsp. celery seed

Remove skin and visible fat from chicken. Put lemon juice in large bowl. Add egg whites and beat until frothy. Add chicken pieces and coat thoroughly. Let stand 10 minutes, mixing occasionally. In another large bowl, mix remaining ingredients for coating. Heat oven 375 degrees. Spray large cookie sheet with non-stick spray. Remove chicken from lemon-egg mixture and roll in coating, covering evenly. Place on baking sheet and bake, turning once, 50 minutes or until chicken no longer appears red inside.

DINNER

LENTILS IN GRAPE JUICE

1 cup green or brown lentils
4 cups white grape juice
1 sprig fresh rosemary or
1 tsp. dried rosemary
1/4 tsp. ground cloves

1 tsp. ground coriander
2 small carrots, thinly sliced
2 med. onions, finely chopped
sea salt
pepper

Place washed lentils in two-quart pot with all other ingredients. Bring to a boil. Lower heat and simmer, loosely covered, until lentils are tender, about 20-30 minutes, stirring occasionally. Add more juice or water if necessary. Finished dish should not be dry. Serves 6.

CHAPTER 55
High Blood Pressure

"In my life, I have suffered many terrible experiences. Some of which actually happened." - Mark Twain

If life is giving you high blood pressure, take a look at the recipes in this book's chapter on stress for meals to help you relax.

Many ailments depend on your blood's ability to deliver nutrients, oxygen and cells to different parts of the body. Good circulation makes the head clear, the muscles strong and the organs resilient. Try these recipes to get your body into circulation.

BREAKFAST

BLACK BEANS

1 lb. black beans, soaked and drained	2 tbsp. olive oil
2 green bell peppers, chopped, divided in half	1 tsp. olive oil
2 green onions, chopped, divided in half	1/4 cup vinegar
3 cloves garlic, chopped, divided	1/4 cup vinegar
1 tsp. oregano	sea salt
1 bay leaf	chopped fresh coriander

Add water to beans to cover generously. Add one bell pepper, one onion, two cloves garlic, oregano and bay leaf. Cook 1-1/2 hours until beans are desired doneness. Heat oils and add remaining bell pepper, onion and garlic. Cook over moderate heat until onion is soft. Add to beans, along with vinegar and salt to taste. Serve hot with coriander garnish. Serves 4-6.

LUNCH

CHICKEN WITH ALMOND PASTE SAUCE

1/4 cup freshly roasted almonds	2 lbs. chicken breast pieces
1-1/2 tsp. cumin seed	2 tbsp. butter
1-1/2 tsp. coriander seed	1 medium onion, sliced
1/4 tsp. sea salt	1 tbsp. grated orange peel
2 tsp. fresh ginger, grated	2 cinnamon sticks

121

| 2 cloves garlic | 1/2 cup light chicken stock |
| 2 tsp. honey | 1 cup whole milk yogurt |

Grind almonds with cumin, coriander, salt, ginger, garlic and honey in blender or food processor or mortar and pestle to form a paste. (If using a blender, use a few tablespoons of stock to facilitate blending.) In large heavy pan brown chicken in butter. Remove chicken and set aside. Put onion in pan and saute until tender. Add almond mixture to onions and fry gently. Add water to keep from burning. Add grated peel, cinnamon sticks and stock. Simmer for 10 minutes. Return chicken to pan and continue to simmer on low heat 15 minutes or to desired doneness. Add yogurt and heat but do not boil. Keep sauce at a simmer until heated thoroughly.

DINNER

BRUSSEL SPROUTS ALA GARREL

1/2 lb. brussel sprouts	1/4 tsp. black pepper
1 tbsp. butter	1/2 cup wheat bread crumbs
1/4 tsp. nutmeg	

Keep brussel sprouts in the freezer overnight. Remove from freezer and let sit in salt water until defrosted. Rinse well. Cook until medium raw. Saute in butter with nutmeg, black pepper and bread crumbs. Serve warm.

CHAPTER 56
Hoarseness

Avoiding hoarseness is simple horse-sense. First of all, don't graze in a wet field, you may catch cold; second of all, don't yell at the top of your lungs for hours at a time. Easy, right?

If you could kick the person responsible for most of your troubles, you wouldn't be able to sit down for a month.

I find myself speaking for hours at a time when I'm making appearances for book signings or on talk shows. So I've only myself to blame when I lose my voice. But I've discovered some very good recipes for hoarseness; and here they are!

BREAKFAST

CHICKEN ONION SOUP

4 quarts chicken stock
1 lb. chicken, diced
1 lb. onion, sliced
6 cloves garlic, pressed
1/8 tsp. nutmeg
2 tbsp. tarragon vinegar
1 tsp. no-MSG soy sauce

1/8 tsp. black pepper
1/8 tsp. cayenne pepper
1/4 cup whole wheat croutons
1/4 cup grated mozzarella cheese
2 tsp. chopped cilantro
2 tsp. chopped green onion

Heat stock in skillet and simmer veal, onion in garlic for 45 minutes. Add nutmeg, vinegar, soy sauce, black pepper and cayenne pepper. Let simmer 15 minutes more. Pour into oven-proof soup bowls and top with cheese and croutons. Top brown in broiler and serve with cilantro and green onion on top.

LUNCH

PASTA PESTO

1/4 cup grated parmesan cheese
4 cloves garlic, pressed
1/4 cup pine nuts
2 cups packed basil leaves

1/4 cup chopped parsley
1/2 cup olive oil
4 cups cooked spinach pasta

Blend cheese, garlic, nuts, basil and parsley in blender or food processor until mixture resembles a coarse paste. Drizzle in oil and mix well. Serve over cooked pasta.

DINNER

LOW-FAT PASTA SALAD

1 stalk celery with leaves	4 cups cooked spinach pasta
1/2 green bell pepper, seeded	1 tbsp. tomato paste
4 green onions	3 tbsp. vinegar
1/2 cucumber, unpeeled	1 tbsp. white grape juice

Chop celery, pepper, green onions and cucumber very fine. Toss chopped vegetables with pasta. Combine tomato paste, vinegar and grape juice. Mix well and toss with pasta mixture. Chill before serving. Serves 4-6.

OTHER

RED SALSA

2 cups chopped fresh tomatoes	2 cloves garlic, pressed
1 four-ounce can green chilies or	juice of 2 lemons
2 fresh green chilies, finely chopped	1 very ripe avocado, finely diced
1 sweet onion, finely chopped	1 tsp. kelp

Blend tomatoes in blender or food processor. Add remaining ingredients. Blend to desired consistency. Makes about four cups.

CHAPTER 57
Hyperactivity

"Never raise your hand to your children - it leaves your midsection unprotected." - Robert Orben

Never assume the worst when it comes to hyperactive children. It may seem like God has somehow deserted you, but there is hope. Allergies to commercial colorings, flavorings and preservatives have been linked to hyperactivity, and many nutrients have found to benefit this behavioral disorder. Start by trying these recipes, as well as eliminating processed food that contain unnatural ingredients.

BREAKFAST

RAISIN MUFFINS

3 cups rolled oats	1/3 cup sesame seed butter
1/2 cup millet flour	1/2 tsp. sea salt
1 cup wheat germ	1/2 cup ground apricot kernels
1 cup bran	1 cup hot water
1/2 cup raisins	

Mix all dry ingredients and raisins. In medium bowl mix sesame butter in hot water. Stir well. Add to raisin mixture and blend well. Let stand ten minutes. Fill buttered muffin pans 2/3 full. Bake 350 degrees until lightly browned, about 30 minutes. Or drop by teaspoonfuls onto lightly greased cookie sheet. Makes two dozen.

LUNCH

LENTILS AND RICE SPANISH STYLE

3/4 cup lentils	1 green bell pepper, finely chopped
1/2 tsp. sea salt	2 tomatoes, peeled and chopped
2 tbsp. olive oil	1 clove garlic, chopped
1 medium onion, finely chopped	3/4 cup brown rice

Cook lentils in water to cover with salt. Simmer, uncovered, about 35 minutes or until fluffy. Set aside. Heat olive oil. Add onion and pepper until onion is soft. Add tomatoes and garlic. Stir well. Add rice and lentils and stir over low heat until liquid is absorbed. Serves 4-6.

DINNER

TURKEY ASPARAGUS ROLL-UPS

> 5 thin slices turkey breast
> 5 tsp. honey mustard
> 5 stalks cooked asparagus

Spread one teaspoon mustard on one slice turkey breast and roll around asparagus stalk. Repeat procedure for each stalk and serve as fun finger food.

CHAPTER 58
Immune System

Your immune system is two things in one: a biochemical military force and a thing of beauty. It is like the world's best-trained, most intelligent, most efficient army for defense. And, in its design, it is an intricate biochemical cathedral combining the most spectacular features of Westminster Abbey, St. Paul's Cathedral and Notre Dame. Without it, we would not survive.

We must respect our immune system, as we honor our God-given body. As I Corinthians 6:19 asks: "Know ye not that your body is temple of the Holy Spirit?" Is it more honoring to God to abuse your body with bad habits and nutrition, or to honor it?

It is important, not only to eat healthful foods, as contained in the following recipes, but to ingest healthful ideals and lifestyles. This thought is beautifully contained in Phillipians 4:8:

> "Finally, brethren, whatsoever things are true;
> whatsoever things are honest;
> whatsoever things are just;
> whatsoever things are pure;
> whatsoever things are lovely;
> whatsoever things are of good rapport;
> if there be any virtue, and if there be any praise,
> think on these things."

BREAKFAST

SEVEN-GRAIN BREAKFAST BOWL

4-1/2 cups water	1/4 cup brown rice
1/4 cup whole oats	2 tbsp. rye grains
1/4 cup barley	2 tbsp. millet
1/4 cup wheat berries	1/4 tsp. salt
1/4 cup buckwheat groats	

Heat water to boiling. Stir in grains and salt. Return to boil. Cover, lower heat and simmer 90 minutes, stirring occasionally. Serves 2-4.

LUNCH

FRUITED POT ROAST

3 tbsp. sesame oil	1-1/2 cups pitted prunes
1 4-5 lb. rump or chuck roast, well-trimmed	
1 red bell pepper, chopped	1-1/2 cups dried apricots
3 medium onions, coarsely chopped	2-4 tbsp. cornstarch,
1/4 tsp. ground cloves	dissolved in 1/4 cup cold water
2 cups apple juice	1/2 cup sesame seeds

Heat oil in Dutch oven or large pot. Add meat and brown on all sides. Add bell pepper, onions, cloves and apple juice. Cover tightly, reduce heat and simmer two hours or until nearly tender or cover and bake 350 degrees 2-1/2 hours. Add prunes and apricots, continue to cook or bake 30 minutes longer. Thicken liquid in pot by adding cornstarch mixture. Cook until thickened, stirring constantly. To serve, spoon over meat and fruit, sprinkle with sesame seeds. Serves 10.

DINNER

MINESTRONE SOUP

1 cup mixed dried beans	1 cup chopped spinach
9 cups water, divided	1 9-1/2 ounce can Italian plum
1 large onion, chopped	tomatoes in tomato juice
2 cloves garlic, pressed	1 cup whole wheat pasta
2 carrots, chopped	1 tsp. dried oregano
1 stalk celery, chopped	1 tsp. salt
4 cups cabbage, chopped	grated parmesan cheese

In large pot, soak beans overnight in four cups water. Drain. Add five cups water and cook one hour or until tender. Add remaining ingredients and cook 20 minutes more, until pasta is tender. Serve hot, sprinkled with parmesan cheese. Serves 6-8.

CHAPTER 59
Impotency

"Those who fail miserably can achieve greatly." - unknown

For many men, eliminating the stress that can cause impotency is a matter of letting go and letting God - of doing what they can and letting God handle the rest before the rest handles them. Stress, bad habits, and poor nutrition are the three most common reasons for impotency.

There are nutritional deficiencies that can cause impotency as well. Zinc, for example. Circulation is important as well. (See the chapter on circulation for some other recipes that help.) About nutrition, a deficiency of zinc is often at the bottom of impotency.

BREAKFAST

EGGS CREOLE

1 tbsp. oil	2 cups tomatoes, peeled & diced
1 small onion, chopped	1/2 tsp. sea salt
1 stalk celery, chopped	1/4 tsp. cayenne
1 green bell pepper, chopped	4 hard boiled eggs, chopped
2 tbsp. whole wheat flour	4 slices whole wheat toast

Heat oil in pan and saute onion, celery and pepper until soft. Stir in flour. Add tomatoes, salt and cayenne. Cook to make a thick sauce. Add eggs, stirring gently to heat through. Serve on whole wheat toast. Serves four.

BREAKFAST COOKIES

3 bananas	1/2 tsp. salt
1 cup chopped dates	1 tbsp. vanilla
1/2 cup chopped nuts	2 cups quick oats

Mash bananas, leaving some chunks. Add dates and nuts. Beat well. Add salt, vanilla and oats. Drop by teaspoonfuls onto ungreased cookie sheet. Bake 25 minutes at 400 degrees. Remove from sheet immediately and cool. Makes one dozen.

LUNCH

GREAT GRATED SALAD

3 cups grated cabbage
2 cups grated carrots
1/2 cup finely chopped broccoli stalks
1/3 cup sesame seeds
1/4 cup olive oil
2 tbsp. wine vinegar
1 tbsp. toasted sesame seeds
1 tsp. sea salt

1 tsp. honey
1/4 tsp. pepper
1/2 avocado, cubed
lemon juice
1 tomato, diced
1/2 cup sliced cucumber
1/2 cup chopped green bell pepper

Sprinkle avocado with lemon juice to prevent browning. In large bowl, combine cabbage, carrots, broccoli and sesame seeds. Mix well and set aside. In small bowl, combine oil, vinegar, toasted sesame seeds, honey, salt and pepper. Blend into cabbage mixture. Divide cabbage mixture into serving plates or bowls. Form into a mound in center. Place avocado, tomato, cucumber and green pepper in rings around the cabbage mound in colorful pattern. Serves four

POT ROAST WITH SAVORY AND SHALLOTS

1 4-5 pound chuck roast, bone-in
whole wheat flour
3 tbsp. vegetable oil
10 green onions, minced
1 bunch summer savory, minced

2 cups beef stock
1/4 cup grape juice
1 tsp. sea salt
dash pepper

Coat roast in flour. Heat oil in pressure cooker or Dutch oven. Brown roast on all sides. Stir in remaining ingredients. Simmer over low heat and cook at 15 pounds of pressure 35 minutes or roast in Dutch oven 2-1/2 hours. Serves 8-10.

DINNER

EGGPLANT SPREAD

1 large eggplant
2 tbsp. olive oil
1 clove garlic, pressed
1/4 cup sliced green onion

1/4 cup diced green bell pepper
1/2 tsp. pepper
1/2 tsp. paprika
1 cup yogurt

Wash and peel eggplant. Dice into 1/8" pieces. Finely chop in blender or food processor. Heat olive oil in large frying pan. Saute eggplant, garlic, onion, bell pepper and pepper five to ten minutes until tender. Remove from heat and pour into medium bowl to cool. After cooled, stir in yogurt and sprinkle on paprika. Spread on crackers.

COLD HERRING PLATTER

4 herring filets   4 hard-boiled eggs
4 slices black bread   8 pickled onions

Serve herring cold on a platter with black bread, sliced hard-boiled eggs and pickled onions. Serves four.

CHAPTER 60
Infertility

"Both tears and sweat are salty, but they render a different result. Tears will get you sympathy, sweat will get you change." - unknown

Listen to my tape on infertility to get the low down on the many reasons and therapies for infertility. But never stop trying. You don't fail until you stop trying. Besides, sex is a great way to get exercise. It's more fun than jogging and doesn't require expensive shoes.

BREAKFAST

COCKY-LEEKY SOUP

1 3-4 lb. chicken	1/2 tsp. white pepper
3 quarts water	1 cup brown rice
2 tsp. sea salt	6-10 leeks

Place chicken in large pot and add water, salt and pepper. Simmer over low heat 90 minutes to two hours or until tender. Remove cooked chicken from pot. Add rice to broth and simmer 20 minutes. While rice cooks, wash leeks carefully. Cut off and discard the tough green part and shred the white part finely. Shred the chicken meat. Add shredded leeks to simmering broth, cook ten minutes. Add chicken and cook through. Serve hot. Serves 6-8.

BROWN RICE BREAKFAST

1 cup brown rice	1 tbsp. honey
1 tbsp. raisins	1/8 tsp. cinnamon
1 tbsp. chopped hazelnuts	

Steam rice. Mix together raisins, hazelnuts, honey and cinnamon. Add brown rice and stir to mix well. Place mixture in buttered baking dish. Cook in preheated 350 degree oven until brown on top.

LUNCH

"DESIRE" FISH WITH CAPERS

1 five pound whole fish, dressed	4 green onions, chopped
1 cup white wine vinegar	1/2 tsp. salt
1/4 cup olive oil	1 tsp. cumin
1 cup water	1 tbsp. grated ginger
1/2 cup fresh dill or fennel or 3 tbsp. dried	1 tsp. capers

Lay fish in large pot and cover with vinegar, oil and water. Fish may be cut in half to accommodate pot. Add dill, green onions, salt, cumin and ginger. Cover and bring to a boil. Lower heat and simmer 30 minutes. Place fish on serving platter, pour poaching liquid over fish and sprinkle capers on top.

PINEAPPLE FISH CASSEROLE

1 lb. flounder filets	1/2 cup pineapple juice
6 slices pineapple	1 egg
2 green onions, chopped	1/2 tsp. salt
2 tsp. cornstarch	

Oil one-quart casserole dish. Preheat oven to 350 degrees. Arrange fish in bottom of dish, top with pineapple slices and green onions. Mix cornstarch with pineapple juice until smooth. Beat in egg and salt. Pour mixture over fish. Bake 30 minutes until lightly brown and fish separates easily with a fork. Serves 4-6.

DINNER

CAULIFLOWER SOUP

1 cauliflower	1 tbsp. chopped parsley
6-8 cups milk	2 tbsp. grated parmesan cheese
1/2 tsp. brewer's yeast	1 egg yolk, beaten
1/4 cup nutmeg	juice of 1/2 lemon
1/4 tsp. black pepper	

Divide cauliflower into small pieces. Place in a deep pot. Add milk to cover cauliflower. Add yeast, nutmeg, black pepper, egg yolk, parmesan cheese, lemon juice and parsley. Mix well. Cover and let simmer 15 minutes or until cauliflower is just tender.

RICE SALAD

1 cup cooked, cold brown rice
2 green onions, chopped
1 green bell pepper, chopped
2 carrots, chopped
1 stalk celery, chopped

1/4 cup real maple syrup
1/2 tsp. cilantro or parsley
1 tbsp. chopped pinenuts
1 tbsp. raisins

Combine all ingredients and serve.

CHAPTER 61
Low Blood Pressure

"I have gained and lost the same ten pounds so many times over and over again my cellulite must have deja vu." - Jane Wagner

Moderation in all things, says the Lord. This includes dieting, one of the reasons for low blood pressure. Women who continually diet to lose weight often forego the nutrients that keep them healthy, and their blood pressure drops. Anything that threatens the body can cause low blood pressure. Anything that nourishes the body will alleviate the problem.

These recipes contain pantothenic acid, protein, the B vitamins and C - valuable warriors in the fight against low blood pressure.

BREAKFAST

POTATO PANCAKES

1/2 onion, finely chopped	1 tsp. lemon juice
1 large unpeeled potato, grated and rinsed	2 tbsp. yogurt
1/3 cup whole wheat cracker crumbs	olive oil
3 tbsp. chopped parsley	

Mix together onion, potato, crumbs, parsley, lemon juice and yogurt. Form four patties with mixture. Cook slowly in oil in hot skillet over moderate heat until brown on both sides. Serve hot.

LUNCH

STUFFED PEPPERS

3/4 cup brown rice	1/2 cup wheat germ
1-1/2 cups vegetable or beef stock	2 tbsp. lemon juice
2 tbsp. vegetable oil	1/2 tsp. ground ginger
1 medium onion, finely chopped	2 tbsp. chopped parsley
1 lb. ground chuck	2 eggs, beaten
1 clove garlic, crushed	1/2 cup broth or water

135

1 tsp. sea salt   6 large sweet red bell peppers
2 tomatoes, peeled, seeded and chopped

Add rice to stock and bring to a boil. Cover and reduce heat. Simmer 20 minutes until rice is tender. Meanwhile, heat oil and saute onion until soft. Add beef and cook until lightly browned. Add garlic. To cooled meat mixture add rice, salt, tomatoes, wheat germ, lemon juice, ginger, parsley and eggs. Cut a thin slice from pepper stems. Stuff with rice-meat mixture. Place peppers, stuffed side up, in large, heavy pot. Add broth, bring to a boil, cover and simmer 30 minutes or until peppers are soft. Add water if necessary.

DINNER

LEEK SOUFFLE

4 leeks   1/8 tsp. cayenne pepper
juice of 1 lime   1/2 tsp. chopped parsley
1/2 tsp. brewer's yeast   1/4 tsp. oregano
1/8 tsp. nutmeg   1 tbsp. parmesan cheese
1/8 tsp. black pepper

Cut leeks in half lengthwise and steam slightly. Place into a buttered baking pan. Sprinkle on yeast, nutmeg, black pepper, cayenne pepper, lime juice, parsley and oregano. Top with parmesan cheese. Let brown in 350 degree oven and serve.

CHAPTER 62
Menopause

Many women are waiting until their later years to have children. Some of them are even going through the change of life and change of diapers at the same time.

Menopause is not the end of a chapter, it's the beginning of a new book! Many, many women are enjoying their "silver" years, and with these recipes, which contain foods rich in the B complex vitamins and vitamin E, menopause needn't be a negative experience.

BREAKFAST

WINTER LENTIL SOUP

1 cup lentils	1 clove garlic, pressed
1-1/2 cup water	1/4 tsp. thyme
1 medium potato, peeled and diced	3 tbsp. no-MSG soy sauce
1 small turnip, peeled and diced	sea salt
1 small carrot, peeled and diced	pepper
1 medium onion, chopped	

Cook lentils in water, covered, 25-30 minutes, until tender but not mushy. In separate large pot, cook potato, turnip and carrot in water 10 minutes or until just tender. Add lentils and any cooking water to vegetables. Mix. Add onion and remaining ingredients including salt and pepper to taste. Simmer 30-40 minutes or until onion is tender and ingredient flavors are well-blended. Serves four.

LUNCH

CHINESE FRIED RICE

2 tbsp. olive oil	1/2 cup fresh or frozen peas
1 tsp. sea salt	1 cup mung bean sprouts
1 medium onion, finely chopped	6 cups cold, cooked brown rice
1 stalk celery, finely chopped	3 tbsp. no-MSG soy sauce
1 cup cooked chicken, diced (optional)	2 green onions, finely chopped
2 eggs, lightly beaten	

Heat oil in wok or very large skillet. Add salt, onion, celery and chicken, if desired. Stir until onion is clear. Mix in eggs, stirring until cooked. Add peas and bean sprouts. Mix well. Add rice and heat thoroughly. Add soy sauce and blend. Garnish with green onions. Serves six.

DINNER

ASPARAGUS IN VINAIGRETTE

2 tbsp. raspberry vinegar
1/2 cup olive oil
1/8 tsp. black pepper
1/8 tsp. white pepper
1/8 tsp. nutmeg

4 cloves garlic, chopped
several mint leaves, crushed
8 stalks cooked asparagus
2 tbsp. wheat germ

In small bowl combine vinegar, oil, peppers, nutmeg and garlic. Add mint leaves and asparagus. Blend well and let soak one hour or more. To serve, top with wheat germ.

CHAPTER 63
Miscarriage

"Life is what happens when you are making other plans." - Woody Allen

Nutrition can make the difference between losing a child and keeping it, many studies have shown. Vitamin E and C have been shown to prevent miscarriages; as well as the bioflavonoid present in citrus fruit peel. If you have a history of miscarriages, avoid stress and practice your cooking with these recipes.

BREAKFAST

HEALTHY BREAKFAST BARS

1 cup cooked millet	1/2 cup sesame seeds
1-1/2 cup dates, finely chopped	1 tsp. vanilla
1 cup shredded coconut	2 tbsp. finely grated orange peel
1 cup almond butter	1 tbsp. finely grated lemon peel
1 cup sorghum	1/2 tsp. sea salt

In large bowl, mix all ingredients well. Use a long wooden spoon and plenty of elbow grease. You may find it easier to blend ingredients with your hands. Shape into two-inch long rolls about an inch wide, wrap in wax paper and chill. Slice into 1/4" thick pieces to serve. Makes about 1-1/2 dozen.

LUNCH

PHAROAH'S DUCK

2 five pound ducks, cut up	4 cups grape juice
sea salt	1/2 cup red wine vinegar
1-1/2 cups barley flour	cayenne

Salt the duck pieces and roll in flour. Bake in 350 degree oven until brown. In large skillet, combine grape juice and vinegar. Add duck and cook over medium heat until tender. Add sea salt and cayenne to taste.

DINNER

ASPARAGUS SALAD

1 lb. asparagus	1/4 tsp. black pepper
1/2 cup tarragon vinegar	1 medium onion, chopped
1/2 cup olive oil	1/2 tsp. chopped parsley
1/8 tsp. nutmeg	1 small clove garlic, chopped
1 tsp. Dijon mustard	1 tbsp. chopped walnuts

Cut asparagus into one-inch pieces and steam. Allow to cool. Add a mixture of vinegar, oil, onion, garlic, parsley, black pepper, nutmeg and Dijon mustard. Add. Let soak at least 30 minutes and serve.

CHAPTER 64
Mononucleosis

My neighbor had to tell her boyfriend she had mono. He thought she meant she had an antique record player.

Mononucleosis has been called the kissing disease because of the high incidence of the flu-like virus among college students in the '80s. It has since been associated with Epstein-Barr Syndrome, and the similar chronic fatigue syndrome.

While vitamin C cannot cure the disease, it can control the severity of the symptoms. These recipes emphasize vitamin C for your quick recovery.

BREAKFAST

BAKED SESAME SEED PEARS

4 firm pears	1 tsp. honey
3 tbsp. currants	1/2 cup apple juice
3 tbsp. sunflower seeds	ground nutmeg
1 tbsp. lemon juice	1/4 cup toasted sesame seeds

Halve and core pears; do not peel them. Place them in an oiled shallow baking dish. Combine currants and sunflower seeds. Stuff in pear halves. Blend lemon juice, honey and juice in bowl. Drizzle over pear halves and dust with nutmeg. Cover and bake at 350 degrees 20 - 30 minutes. To serve, garnish with sesame seeds.

LUNCH

BRUSSEL SPROUT CHICKEN SOUP

1 lb. brussel sprouts	1 clove garlic
1 chicken	1/2 tsp. black pepper
4 qts. chicken stock	1/4 tsp. cayenne pepper
2 leeks	1/8 tsp. nutmeg
2 onions	1/8 tsp. chopped parsley/serving
4 carrots	

Steam brussel sprouts until tender. Skin the chicken, and combine all ingredients in large cooking pot. Simmer until tender. Top with chopped parsley before serving.

DINNER

VEGETABLES VINAIGRETTE

1/2 cup two-inch carrot sticks	1 tsp. sea salt
1/2 cup two-inch celery sticks	1/4 tsp. freshly ground pepper
1/2 cup asparagus tips	1/2 clove garlic, pressed
1/2 cup green onion bulbs	2 tbsp. wine vinegar
1/2 cup small mushroom caps	1/2 cup olive oil

Cook carrots, celery, asparagus and green onions separately in boiling, salted water until just tender. Drain, rinse thoroughly in cold water and drain again. Place cooked vegetables and mushroom caps in glass bowl. Set aside. Put salt, pepper and garlic in small bowl. Mash together thoroughly. Add vinegar and stir until salt dissolves. Stir in oil. Pour vinaigrette into bowl with vegetables. Cover and refrigerate overnight. To serve, toss, drain and arrange on serving platter.

CHAPTER 65
Motion Sickness

"One of the best temporary cures for pride and affectation is seasickness; a man who wants to vomit never puts on airs. - Josh Billings (1818-1882)

For some people, just the thought of riding in the backseat of a car on a long, winding road brings on pangs of nausea.

Goodbye motion sickness, hello ginger root!

Double-blind tests have shown eating ginger can ease the queasiness of motion or sea sickness, and even morning sickness among pregnant women. Since ginger can burn when eaten raw, instead try these recipes that contain it.

BREAKFAST

GINGERED WHEAT BREAD

3 cups water	1/4 cup vegetable oil
1/2 cup honey	1 cup wheat germ
1/4 tsp. ground ginger	2 tsp. salt
6 pkgs. dry yeast	10 cups unsifted whole wheat flour

Heat water to 115 degrees. Keep all other ingredients at room temperature. Mix honey and ginger with warm water. Stir in yeast, cover and let stand in warm place for ten minutes, until frothy. Add oil, wheat germ and salt. Mix in five cups of flour. Add flour gradually, mixing with hands to make a fairly stiff dough. Turn the dough out onto a well-floured board and knead until smooth and elastic. Add flour as needed.

Place dough in well-oiled bowl and turn dough to cover with oil. Cover and put into warm place to rise. The dough should double in 45 minutes. When doubled, punch the dough down. Turn punched side to bottom of bowl. Cover and let rise again for about 30 minutes. Turn the dough onto a floured board and let stand ten minutes. Divide into thirds and shape into three loaves. Place loaves into well-oiled loaf pans. Cover and let rise until nearly doubled. Bake at 350 degrees for 40 minutes or until crust is brown and makes a hollow noise when you tap it.

LUNCH

APRICOT GINGER PASTA SALAD

16 dried apricot halves
1/4 cup chopped walnuts
2 cups cooked wheat and spinach pasta
1-1/2 tbsp. olive oil

1 tbsp. lemon juice
1/2 tbsp. grated lemon peel
1/4 tsp. ground ginger
dash cayenne

Soak apricots in water ten minutes. Drain and slice. Combine apricots, walnuts and pasta. In separate bowl, combine remaining ingredients. Pour over apricot mixture and toss to mix. Serve cold or at room temperature.

DINNER

GINGERED PAPAYA

4 firm, ripe papayas
8 tbsp. butter, divided
4 tbsp. lime juice, divided

1 tsp. ground ginger, divided
8 thin slices lime
dash cayenne

Preheat oven to 350 degrees. Cut papayas in half, lengthwise. Scoop out seeds. Arrange in glass baking dish with 1/8" warm water in bottom. In each papaya hollow, place 1 tbsp. butter, 1/2 tbsp. lime juice and 1/8 tsp. ground ginger. Bake 30 minutes, basting 10 minutes before done. Place a slice of lime at corner of each papaya half before serving. Top with sprinkle of cayenne. Serve warm.

OTHER

GINGER TEA

1/4 tsp. ground ginger
1 cup hot water

1 tsp. honey
1 tsp. lemon juice

Stir ginger in hot water. Add honey and lemon to taste.

WATERMELON GINGER

1/2 watermelon, cut into bite-sized chunks
1/2 cup grape juice

1 tbsp. honey
2 pieces candied ginger, grated

In saucepan combine grape juice, water and honey. Heat gently on low heat. Remove from heat and add ginger. Let cool. Pour mixture over watermelon. Refrigerate for several hours.

CHAPTER 66
Osteoporosis
(How to have brawny bones)

Age is all in how you look at it. If you don't care how old you are, you're young. When you lie about how old you are, you're middle aged. And if you brag about how old you are, you're a senior citizen taking advantage of discounts.

Osteoporosis is not a necessary evil of old age. It can be prevented and even, to some degree, cured. Don't let your shell become brittle and bent, use these recipes to keep your bones brawny and your marrow mighty.

BREAKFAST

PEAR AND GRAPE COMPOTE

2 pears, diced
1 lb. seedless grapes, sliced in half
1/2 cup *real maple syrup
3 dried mint flakes

juice of 1/2 lemon
1/4 tsp. cinnamon
cooked barley

Mix ingredients together in a saucepan and cook for 10 minutes. Serve over barley.

*Note: pure maple syrup is high in calcium, potassium and phosphorous, nutrients vital to your bones, and should not be mistaken for food-free maple-flavored syrup.

HEAVENLY HERRING

4 herring filets approximately 4 " long
1 cup watercress, stems removed
1 orange, peeled, cut into thin slices

1/4 tsp. black pepper
1/2 red onion, cut into thin slices

Separate watercress into small leaf clusters. Cut herring into half pieces, reserving a filet to cut into longer lengths for garnish. Arrange herring pieces, watercress clusters and orange and onion slices into equal portions on four salad plates.

dressing:

2 tbsp. orange juice	1/4 cup champagne vinegar
1 tbsp. chopped shallots	1/8 tsp. black pepper
1/3 cup olive oil	

Combine dressing ingredients until thickened. Pour over each salad. Garnish with reserved herring strips crisscrossing them over the contents of each plate.

LUNCH

GREEN SALAD SPECIAL

2 heads butter lettuce	1/4 tsp. nutmeg
1/2 cup tarragon vinegar	1 tbsp. honey
1/4 cup half and half	1/4 cup chopped walnuts
1/4 cup diced green apple	1/4 cup raisins
1/4 cup medium yellow onion, sliced	1 cup cottage cheese
1 tsp. chopped dill	1 tbsp. lemon juice
1 tsp. chopped parsley	1/4 cup tomato juice
1/2 tsp. black pepper	1 hard boiled egg, finely chopped

Rinse and dry lettuce well. Place lettuce in a large bowl and mix with remaining ingredients. Decorate with sprinkles of chopped walnuts and raisins. In blender or food processor, blend cottage cheese and lemon juice. Add tomato juice and blend until very smooth. Add more tomato juice if necessary. Stir egg into dressing just before serving. Toss with salad or serve on the side.

SUCCULENT SALMON STEAK

2 tsp. olive oil	1/2 bunch cilantro, chopped
4 four-ounce salmon steaks	1 tbsp. fresh grated ginger root
12 green onions, cut lengthwise	

Grease large stainless steel cookie sheet with olive oil. Place salmon steaks on sheet. Cover steaks with green onions, cilantro and ginger. Cover with foil. Bake in 350 degree oven 25-30 minutes or barbecue over hot coals.

DINNER

DATE-NUT SPREAD

1 cup pitted dates	1/4 cup non-instant powdered milk
1/2 cup chopped pistachios	celery stalks, cut into 2" pieces
1/4 cup yogurt	

Puree dates, nuts, yogurt and powdered milk in blender or food processor. Add more dried milk if it is too thin to spread. Serve spread on celery stalks.

CAULIFLOWER AU GRATIN

1 large cauliflower	pepper
2 eggs	1/2 cup grated parmesan cheese
2/3 cup skim milk	2 tbsp. butter
sea salt	

Preheat oven to 450 degrees. Break cauliflower into florets and steam in small amount of boiling water until barely tender. Drain and mash coarsely. Whisk together eggs and milk, and add to cauliflower. Mix well. Salt and pepper to taste. Place mixture in lightly buttered 1-1/2 quart casserole dish. Sprinkle with cheese and dot with butter. Bake in 450 degree oven for 20 minutes.

CHAPTER 67
PMS

In France I saw a quaint sight: a man walking toward me with a loaf of bread tucked under his arm. Unfortunately, he was my waiter.
- *Current Comedy*

Endure no longer - the solution to premenstrual syndrome's trials is at hand! Good nutrition and exercise can be the light at the end of the PMS tunnel. Avoid processed foods, salt, and concentrate on healthy food fare such as the meals shown here.

BREAKFAST

AVOCADO PIE

crust:
 butter
 1 lb. pitted dates, mashed
 1/2 cup ground walnuts
 1/4 cup shredded coconut
 4 tbsp. coconut juice

filling:
 3 medium ripe avocados
 1/2 cup crushed pineapple
 6 tbsp. coconut juice
 5 tbsp. pure maple syrup
 3 tbsp. apple pectin
 3 tbsp. pineapple juice
 1 kiwifruit, peeled and sliced

Lightly grease a 9" pie pan with butter. Combine crust ingredients and blend until mixture is a soft dough. Press mixture into pie pan, making sure crust is evenly distributed. Cover and refrigerate. In medium bowl, mash avocados. Add pineapple, coconut juice and syrup. Heat pineapple juice to boiling, add apple pectin, lower heat, and stir until thickened. Add to filling mixture and mix well. Pour into chilled pie crust and refrigerate thoroughly before serving.

POTATO LEEK SOUP

 1 lb. potatoes
 4 qts. chicken or vegetable stock
 4 leeks, whole
 1 whole clove garlic
 2 medium yellow onions

 1 tsp. ground black pepper
 1/2 tsp. cayenne pepper
 1/4 tsp. nutmeg
 chopped parsley

Dice potatoes, leeks, onions, and garlic and place all ingredients in a pot. Simmer over medium heat until potatoes are tender. Decorate with cilantro or parsley.

LUNCH

POTATO SALAD

4 large baking potatoes, scrubbed
1 tsp. chopped parsley
2 tbsp. chopped red onion
1/4 cup chopped green bell pepper
1/4 cup chopped black olives
freshly ground black pepper

cayenne
3-1/2 tbsp. mayonnaise
1 tbsp. mustard
1 tbsp. and 1 tsp. cider vinegar
4 hard boiled eggs, chopped

Cut potatoes in 1/2" cubes and boil until just done, about 10 minutes. Drain and reserve cooking water. Chill. Toss chilled potatoes with parsley, onion. bell peppers, pepper and cayenne to taste. Add mayonnaise and mustard to potatoes, blend well. Add vinegar and stir to mix thoroughly. Carefully blend in eggs last. For best results, let chill overnight prior to serving.

HERBED HEALTH SALAD

salad:
1/2 ripe avocado, sliced
1/2 cucumber, sliced
1 cup mung sprouts
1 cup sliced summer squash
1 cup ground apricot kernels
2 tbsp. sunflower seeds
1 cup chopped spinach
1/8 cup olive oil
1 tomato, quartered
1/2 red bell pepper, seeded and sliced

herb dressing:
1 tsp. kelp
1/4 tsp. freshly ground pepper
1/2 clove garlic, pressed
1/2 tbsp. marjoram flowers
1/2 tbsp. freshly ground mint
2 tbsp. wine vinegar
1/2 cup olive oil

Mix salad ingredients together in large bowl. Set aside. Put kelp, pepper, garlic, marjoram and mint in small bowl. Mash together thoroughly. Add vinegar and stir until salt dissolves. Stir in oil. For best results, place in jar and allow to marinate overnight in refrigerator. Shake jar and pour herb dressing over salad ingredients. Toss wel¹ before serving.

DINNER

POTATO SOUFFLE

4 medium potatoes, diced	1/4 tsp. nutmeg
2 medium onions, chopped	4 bay leaves, crumbled
1/4 cup parsley, chopped	1/2 cup wheat bread crumbs
1/4 cup dill, chopped	1/4 cup grated parmesan cheese
1/2 tsp. black pepper	1/4 cup cold butter

Combine potato, onion, parsley, dill and bay leaves in a buttered souffle dish. Over top sprinkle pepper, nutmeg, bread crumbs, parmesan cheese and bits of crumbled butter. Bake for 45 min. at 375 degrees.

COUNTRY CORNBREAD

1 cup whole wheat flour	2 tbsp. honey
3/4 cup yellow cornmeal	1 egg, beaten
2 tsp. baking powder	2/3 cup yogurt
1/2 tsp. salt	1/4 cup olive oil

Preheat oven to 425 degrees. Oil an 8" square baking pan. Stir dry ingredients together. Stir liquid ingredients together and blend into dry ingredients, little by little; stirring after each addition until batter is moist. Do not overmix. Pour into pan and bake 20-25 minutes.

CHAPTER 68
Prenatal

For I will pour water upon him that is thirsty, and floods upon dry ground: I will pour my spirit upon thy seed, and my blessing upon thine offspring. - Isaiah 44:3

In honor of the unborn, do everything possible to ensure a strong and healthy beginning. Several nutrients have been shown to have "bearing" upon the health of the unborn child. They are vitamins B6, E, folic acid, magnesium and zinc. The recipes contained here were specially conceived with this principle in mind.

BREAKFAST

CURRIED EGGS

2 tbsp. oil	1 cup milk
1 carrot, grated	1 tbsp. lemon juice
1 onion, finely chopped	sea salt
1 apple, grated	6 hard boiled eggs, chopped
2 tbsp. whole wheat flour	whole grain bread
1 tbsp. curry powder	

Heat oil and saute carrot, onion and apple until soft. Stir in flour and curry. Gradually stir in milk. Cook about five minutes or until sauce thickens. Add lemon juice and salt to taste. Add eggs and heat through. Serve over whole grain toast.

ZUCCHINI BREAD

2 eggs	1 cup water
1 cup honey	1 cup olive oil
1/2 cup blackstrap molasses	2 cups grated zucchini
grated rind and juice of 1 lemon	1 cup apricots, chopped
2-1/2 cups whole wheat flour	1 cup slivered almonds
2 tsp. baking powder	

Beat eggs. Add honey and molasses while beating. Add rind and lemon juice. In separate bowl, mix flour and baking powder together. Add water and oil alternately to flour. Add egg mixture, zucchini and apricots. Place in 9" x 13" baking dish. Sprinkle top with almonds. Bake in 350 degree oven 40-45 minutes.

LUNCH

HEALTHY BABY BULGUR SALAD

1 cup fine-grained bulgur	sea salt to taste
3 cups boiling water	3 tbsp. olive oil
1 bunch green onions, finely chopped	1 tsp. prepared sharp mustard
2 cups chopped parsley	Romaine lettuce leaves
4 tbsp. vinegar or lemon juice	2 cloves garlic, chopped
1/2 cup chopped radishes	

In a large bowl, cover bulgur with boiling water; soak 30 minutes or until tender. Drain and combine all ingredients except lettuce leaves. Chill several hours or overnight. Serving: Arrange lettuce leaves in a circle on a platter and put salad in center.

STUFFED SAVOY CABBAGE

1 large Savoy cabbage	1/2 tsp. thyme
1 large square of cheesecloth	1/4 tsp. basil
1 pound ground chuck	sea salt
1 large onion, finely chopped	pepper
1 clove garlic, pressed	2 tbsp. vegetable oil
4 tsp. tomato paste	2 large carrots, sliced
1/2 cup cooked millet	1 large onion, sliced
1 egg	3 cups water

Cook the whole cabbage in boiling salted water to cover 10 to 15 minutes. Drain and rinse with cold water. Allow to cool. Remove very tough or discolored outer leaves. Place cabbage, stem side down, on cheesecloth. Gently pry leaves apart and cut out the core, leaving stem intact. Mix together meat, onion, garlic, tomato paste, millet, egg, thyme, basil, salt and pepper. Place mixture into hollowed cabbage. Gently push leaves back, reshaping the cabbage. Tie cheesecloth firmly around cabbage. Heat oil in large pan. Saute carrots and onion, then add water and cabbage. Cover and simmer 2-1/2 to 3 hours. Remove cheesecloth before serving. Serves 6.

DINNER

HUMUS

1-1/2 cups dried chickpeas
3 cloves garlic, pressed
1/2 cup sesame tahini
juice of 1 lemon
1 tsp. sea salt

parsley
lemon wedges
paprika
whole wheat bread sticks

In large saucepan cover chickpeas in water. Bring to a boil and cook three minutes. Cover and let stand one hour. Drain and reserve liquid. Mash chickpeas. Set aside. Combine garlic with tahini. Add lemon juice and salt. Mix well. Grind mashed chickpeas in blender or food processor a little at a time, adding tahini mixture and chickpea cooking water as needed. Humus should be thick. Garnish with parsley and lemon wedges. Sprinkle with paprika and serve with or on whole wheat sesame crackers.

SPROUT SALAD

3 cups alfalfa sprouts, rinsed and dried
2 slices pineapple, diced
1 apple, diced
1/4 cup chopped cilantro
1/4 cup green onions, diced

1/2 pound grapes
1/4 cup pinenuts
1/4 cup raspberry vinegar
1/2 tsp. black pepper

Mix ingredients together and serve.

CHAPTER 69
Prostrate Problems

. "If the world were a logical place, men would ride sidesaddle." - Rita Mae Brown

When your prostrate is growing faster than your bank balance, it's time to consider nutrition to battle this common male ailment.

There's something about the prostate gland that makes it susceptible to all sorts of disorders from infections to enlargement to cancer. Why does age have to include prostatitis? It doesn't!

Please your prostrate with low-fat, whole foods high in zinc and essential fatty acids, like the ones in these recipes.

BREAKFAST

GRIDDLE CAKES

2 cups soaked soy beans, pureed	1 tsp. salt
1 cup water	2/3 cup whole wheat flour
1 cup skim milk	2/3 cup millet flour
1 tsp. honey	warm pure maple syrup

Combine all ingredients except flours and syrup in bowl. Mix well and add flours, a little at a time until well blended. Spoon onto medium hot griddle. Brown both sides and serve with pure maple syrup.

LUNCH

FELAFEL

patties:

1/4 cup bulgur	1/4 tsp. black pepper
2 cups cooked garbanzos, mashed	1/4 tsp. turmeric
2 cloves garlic, pressed	1/4 tsp. coriander
3 tbsp. whole wheat bread crumbs	1 tbsp. chopped parsley
1 egg, beaten	1/8 tsp. cayenne pepper
1/2 tsp. sea salt	olive oil
1/2 tsp. cumin	

whole wheat pita bread.

tahini dressing:
1 cup lemon juice	1/2 cup chopped parsley
1 cup yogurt	1/4 tsp. cayenne
1 cucumber, diced	sea salt
1 tomato, peeled and diced	pepper

To make felafel patties, mix together all ingredients and chill. Shape into patties and fry in oil until golden brown. Place hot patties in pita pocket with combined dressing ingredients.

DINNER

LIMA-RICE CHOWDER

1 cup dried lima beans	1/4 tsp. dried thyme
1 medium onion, finely chopped	4 tbsp. chopped fresh parsley
1 red bell pepper, diced	1/2 cup raw brown rice
1 green bell pepper, diced	2 tbsp. sesame tahini
2 carrots, diced	1/4 cup no-MSG soy sauce
2 stalks celery, diced	dash cayenne pepper
4 cloves garlic, pressed	

Rinse lima beans and discard any that are discolored. Soak overnight in water to cover; drain. Add water to limas to generously cover and bring to a boil. Lower heat; simmer one hour, or until beans are soft. Add onion, peppers, carrots, celery, garlic, thyme, parsley and rice to limas. Add water to cover by about two inches. Bring to a boil. Cover and simmer over low heat 30 minutes, or until rice is tender. Stir in tahini sauce and soy sauce. Add cayenne to taste and thin with water, if necessary. Serves four to six.

CHAPTER 70
Psoriasis

An imperfection which humbles a person is of more value to him than a deed which feeds his ego.

Pharmaceutical companies like to make you believe an ailment is worse than it is, so you look to them for a cure or relief. The "heartbreak of psoriasis," was used in advertising to make people think of psoriasis as a tragic disease.

As long ago as the 1600s, people were not fooled by conventional medicine. Voltaire, a 15th century writer, is quoted as having said, "The art of medicine consists of amusing the patient while nature cures the disease."

The irony is that oftentimes stress from an emotional or physical upheaval can bring on a case of psoriasis. Cold water fish and lecithin has shown to work wonders in treating psoriasis. Try these recipes and you may be pleasantly surprised to discover your heart has mended.

BREAKFAST

BARLEY CAROB CAKE

2 eggs, beaten	1 cup and 2 tbsp. barley flour
3/4 cup honey	1/2 cup safflower oil
1/2 cup carob flour	3/4 cup water
2-1/2 tsp. baking powder	1 tsp. vanilla

Combine honey and eggs. Mix well. Mix carob, baking powder and flour. Combine two mixtures. Add oil and water alternately. Add vanilla and blend well. Pour into an 8" x 8" oiled baking pan and bake 300 degrees until toothpick inserted into center comes out clean, about 40 minutes. Cool about five minutes then remove and cool on rack.

LUNCH

HERBED SALMON FILET

4 salmon filets
1 tbsp. olive oil
1/2 tsp. black pepper
1/4 tsp. cayenne pepper
1/4 cup chopped dill

1/4 tsp. oregano
1/4 cup honey
juice of 1/2 lime
1/4 cup sliced almonds

Skin, clean, and dry salmon filets. In small bowl mix all other ingredients except almonds. Place fish in baking pan and pour sauce on top. Sprinkle almonds on top and bake in 375-degree oven approximately 15 minutes.

DINNER

BEET AND HERRING SALAD

4 medium herring filets
2 cups sour cream
2 medium beets, cooked
1 tsp. ground cloves

1 tsp. chopped dill
1/2 tsp. black pepper
1/2 tsp. rosemary

Rinse herring filets well in cold water. Spread one cup sour cream in serving dish. Cut beets into small slices and place on top. In small bowl, combine rest of sour cream, cloves, dill, pepper and rosemary. Mix well. Place herring over beets and cover with herb mixture. Allow to sit for 1 hour or more before serving to develop flavor.

CHAPTER 71
Shingles

"Dogs come when they're called. Cats take a message and get back to you." - Mary Bly

What do shingles have to do with cats? Nothing, I just thought this was funny. What do shingles have to do with chickens? Plenty, when you're talking about chicken pox and herpes zoster, which is the medical name for shingles.

It turns out, the same virus that causes chicken pox in children, turns around and gives adults shingles, even if they've had the pox already. But help is at hand!

Foods high in vitamin B12, C and E can end the pain and discomfort of shingles. For tasty, pox-ending meals, try these recipes.

BREAKFAST

SUPER GRANOLA

2 cups rolled oats	1/3 cup chopped cashews
2 cups rolled wheat	1/3 cup chopped walnuts
1 cup shredded coconut	1/3 cup chopped almonds
1/2 cup sesame seeds	1/3 cup sunflower seeds
1/2 cup wheat germ	2 cups raisins
1/2 cup date sugar	1/2 cup non-instant powdered milk
1/2 cup toasted peanut flour (optional)	

Mix all ingredients together. Store tightly covered in refrigerator. Makes about nine cups.

LUNCH

APRICOT ZUCCHINI SOUFFLE

16 dried apricot halves
4 eggs, separated
3/4 cup grated zucchini

1/2 tsp. cinnamon
dash Spike

Soak dried apricots overnight. Mash 12 of the apricots with a fork. Cut remaining four into 1/4" cubes. Preheat oven to 350 degrees. In large bowl, beat egg yolks. Stir in apricots, zucchini and cinnamon. Whip egg whites with Spike until stiff peaks form. Carefully fold into apricot mixture. Pour into greased two-quart souffle dish or 8" x 8" baking pan. Bake 30-40 minutes or until puffed and lightly brown. Serve immediately.

DINNER

PUMPKIN KLARA

1 2-pound pumpkin
juice of 1/2 lemon
1/4 tsp. black pepper

1/4 cup honey mustard
Belgian endive
raspberry vinegar

Peel and slice pumpkin into french fry-sized pieces. Mix together lemon, pepper and honey mustard. Place pumpkin in skillet with lemon mixture. Simmer over low heat 15 minutes or until pumpkin is tender. Serve with thinly-sliced Belgian endive sprinkled with raspberry vinegar.

CHAPTER 72
Skin, Hair and Nails

"Not every woman in old slippers can look like Cinderella." - Don Marquis

Before you reach for the hair dye consider these words of wisdom: "Gray hairs seem to my fancy like the soft light of the moon, silvering over the evening of life." - Richter

When I fed my hair (and the rest of me) junk food, I lost hair in handfuls. It was my hairdresser, Karl Rolfes, who told me "If I was your hair I would have left home a long time ago." With the secret of nutrition, I now have thick, lustrous hair.

Skin, hair and nails are all pretty much governed by the same nutritional needs, which is why they end up lumped together. Nails are basically compacted hair. Another thing they have in common: a problem with them can indicate an underlying, more serious condition.

Use these recipes to keep your skin, hair and nails looking their best. But get my audio tapes on skin, hair and nails for more thorough information. Call or write 1-800-445-HEAL or read my book *Foods That Heal*, available at Box 844, Menlo Park, CA 94026.

BREAKFAST

CARROT BREAD

1/4 cup molasses	1/2 cup wheat germ
3 cups carrot juice	1/2 cup gluten flour
3 pkgs. dry yeast	8 cups whole wheat flour
2 tsp. sea salt	2 cups grated carrots
3 tbsp. vegetable oil	

Add molasses to carrot juice, stir in yeast, cover and let stand 10 minutes or until yeast is bubbly. Add salt and oil to yeast mixture. Mix wheat germ and gluten flour with five cups of whole wheat flour. Add mixture to yeast and beat well. Cover with cloth and let rise 10 minutes. Stir in carrots and add flour, one cup at a time until dough is workable. Knead on a floured board 10 minutes and place dough in oiled bowl, turning to oil dough. Cover and let rise about 45 minutes or until doubled.

Punch dough down. Turn out on floured board and let stand 10 minutes. Meanwhile, oil three loaf pans. Knead dough three to four times and form three loaves. Place loaves seam side down in pans; cover and let rise 45 minutes. During the last ten minutes of rise, heat oven to 375 degrees. Bake 20 minutes, then lower the heat to 300 degrees and bake 30 minutes longer or until done. Remove from pans and cool on wire racks.

RICE SALAD MEDITERRANEAN

1 cup cooked brown rice	3 tbsp. chopped parsley
1 small zucchini, chopped	1 tbsp. capers
1 tbsp. red onion, chopped	1/4 cup olive oil
1 ripe tomato, chopped	1 clove garlic, pressed
1 small red bell pepper, chopped	juice of 1/2 lemon

Mix rice with vegetables, parsley and capers. Combine olive oil and garlic and toss with rice mixture. Add lemon juice and mix well. Serves four.

LUNCH

SWEET POTATO CASSEROLE

3 lbs. fresh or canned sweet potatoes	1 tsp. sea salt
3 eggs, separated	1 cup skim milk
1 tbsp. melted butter	1/4 cup slivered almonds

Mash cooked sweet potatoes. Add well-beaten egg yolks, melted butter, salt and milk. Fold in well-beaten egg whites. Butter three-quart casserole dish. Pour sweet potato mixture in dish and top with almonds. Bake at 325 degrees 20-25 minutes. Serves 6-8.

LIZ'S CHICKEN

4-6 chicken breasts, skin removed	juice of 1/2 lemon
2 tbsp. vegetable oil	2 cups tomato sauce
1 large onion, sliced	3 tbsp. chicken stock
2 cloves garlic, crushed	1/2 tsp. basil
1/2 lb. mushrooms, sliced	1 tbsp. tomato paste
1 carrot, grated	

Saute chicken breasts in oil until lightly browned. Remove chicken from pan and set aside. Add onion, garlic, mushrooms and carrot to the pan and saute until vegetables are limp. Add lemon juice. Cover pan and simmer five minutes. Add tomato sauce, stock and basil, and mix well. Return chicken breasts to pan; cover and simmer on low heat 20 minutes or until chicken is tender. Remove chicken to warm platter. Add tomato paste to sauce mixture and cook, stirring, over high heat until sauce is thickened. Serve over chicken. Serves 4-6.

DINNER

CABBAGE WITH RAISINS

1/2 cup raisins	pinch cinnamon
1/2 cup apple or grape juice	pinch nutmeg
1 large red cabbage	pinch rosemary
2 tbsp. vinegar	sea salt
1 tsp. honey	pepper

Soak raisins in fruit juice at least two hours. Cut cabbage into strips, discarding tough inner core. Oil 13" x 9" baking pan and place cabbage in it. Sprinkle with vinegar. Cover and bake at 350 degrees for 30 minutes. Add raisins, juice, honey, cinnamon, nutmeg and rosemary. Bake another 15 minutes, more if a softer texture is preferred. Salt and pepper to taste.

RED AND YELLOW TOMATO SOUFFLE

5 small red tomatoes	1/4 tsp. nutmeg
5 small yellow tomatoes	1/4 tsp. black pepper
1/4 cup onion, chopped	1/4 tsp. basil
1/4 tsp. paprika	1/4 cup grated parmesan cheese

Slice tomatoes into thin slices and place them into an oiled 13" x 9" baking pan. Surround tomato slices with diced onion. Combine paprika, nutmeg, black pepper basil and parmesan cheese, and sprinkle mixture on top of tomatoes. Bake in 350 degree oven 20 minutes or until tomatoes are cooked and top is light brown.

CHAPTER 73
Sleeplessness

I've discovered that exercise helps me sleep. I keep nodding off in aerobics class.

The first thing to keep in mind about insomnia is not to lose sleep over it. It's a vicious circle: worrying about losing sleep, watching the clock tick by. Instead, have a banana, some lettuce and chamomile tea - and relax! These recipes have foods that contain tryptophan, nature's relaxant.

Come unto Me ye that labor and are heavy laden and I will give you rest. - Psalm 34:15

BREAKFAST

BARLEY FRUIT MUFFINS

1/2 cup shredded apple	1 cup millet flour
3/4 cup water	1/2 tsp. sea salt
1/4 cup vegetable oil	1/2 cup raisins
1 cup barley flour	

Combine apple, oil and water. Set aside. Combine flours and salt. Combine apple mixture and flour mixture. Mix well. Add raisins. Spoon into oiled muffin tins or use paper cups. Bake in 350 degree oven 20 minutes. Makes one dozen.

OATMEAL

2 cups oatmeal	2 tsp. honey
2 tsp. raisins	1/4 tsp. cinnamon
1 banana, chopped	

Cook oatmeal with banana. Place into a buttered baking dish, and pour honey and sprinkle cinnamon on top. Place in 350 degree preheated oven and allow to brown.

<u>LUNCH</u>

BASIC CHEESE SOUFFLE

1 tbsp. grated parmesan cheese	4 egg yolks
3 tbsp. butter	1/2 cup grated cheddar cheese
1/4 cup whole wheat flour	4 egg whites
sea salt	1/2 tsp. sea salt
white pepper	1/2 tsp. cream of tartar

Heat oven to 375 degrees. Oil a 1-1/2 quart souffle mold or charlotte mold. Sprinkle with parmesan cheese. Melt butter in a large saucepan. Add flour and mix. Stir in milk and salt and pepper to taste. Cook, stirring constantly, until sauce is thick and smooth. Remove from heat. Stir in egg yolks, one at a time, mixing well. Add the cheese. Beat egg whites with salt. Add cream of tarter to form stiff peaks. Stir 1/4 of the beaten whites into the yolk mixture. Fold in remaining whites. Pour mixture into souffle mold. Smooth the top. Bake 35-40 minutes or until souffle is puffed and golden.

STUFFED CHICKEN BREASTS

4 chicken breasts, boned and skinned	1/4 tsp. thyme
2 tbsp. brown rice cake crumbs	1/4 tsp. sage
1 stalk celery, with leaves, finely chopped	1 egg white
1 tart apple, cored and finely chopped	1 tbsp. lemon juice
1/2 medium onion, finely chopped	1/2 cup sliced almonds
2 brown rice cakes, finely chopped	

Preheat oven to 325 degrees. Spray inside of four ovenproof one-cup molds with non-stick spray. Set a kettle of water to boil. Place chicken breasts between sheets of waxed paper and pound thin (about 1/4" thick). Sprinkle rice crumbs evenly one side of each chicken breast. Shake off excess. Drape breasts, crumb side down, in prepared baking dishes, allowing any excess to hang over sides. Combine celery, apple and onion. Add rice cakes. Stir in thyme, sage, egg white and lemon juice. Add almonds. Divide mixture into fourths and place on chicken breasts in cups. Fold over excess chicken and bake 350 degrees for 40 minutes or until chicken is brown.

DINNER

TOMATO ASPIC

1 bar agar-agar	juice of 1/2 lemon
4 cups tomato juice	2 sprigs parsley
1 celery stalk, chopped	1 sprig basil
1 onion, chopped	pinch cinnamon
1 carrot, chopped	

In large saucepan, soak agar-agar in tomato juice until soft. Add remaining ingredients. Simmer over low heat, covered, 20 minutes. Strain. Let cool slightly. Pour into chilled mold. Chill until set. Unmold aspic to serve.

BANANA EGG PLANT

1 banana, sliced lengthwise	1/2 tsp. brewer's yeast
1 medium eggplant, sliced	1/4 cup honey
1/2 cup sour cream	1 tsp. mint flakes
1/8 tsp. nutmeg	1 tsp. raisins
1/8 tsp. black pepper	1 tsp. chopped walnuts

Steam or saute eggplant slices until soft. In small bowl combine sour cream, yeast, honey, nutmeg and pepper. Pour mixture into a shallow baking pan. Layer egg plant slices then put banana on top of mixture. Add mint flakes, raisins and walnuts on top. Broil in oven until banana is brown.

CHAPTER 74
Smell/Taste Loss

Common sense is the sixth sense God gave us to keep us from making fools of ourselves with the other five.

While you might not miss the unique and unforgettable experience of a dead skunk on the road, certain smells and tastes are important to your health and safety.

Studies have shown that certain nutrients, especially zinc, can make or break your senses.

BREAKFAST

CAROB BREAD

3 cups barley flour	1 tsp. anise seed
3 cups whole wheat flour	1 tsp. pepper
1/2 cup carob flour	pinch cumin
2 tbsp. vegetable oil	2 tbsp. toasted sesame seeds
2 tsp. cinnamon	1 tbsp. poppy seeds
1 tsp. nutmeg	1 cup yogurt
4 tbsp. honey	warm water

Combine all ingredients into a dough. Knead dough at least ten minutes. Shape into two loaves and place into oiled 9" x 5" loaf pans. Let rise three hours, reshaping if necessary. Carob must be baked at low temperature to prevent burning. Preheat oven to 300 degrees. Place a pan of warm water next to loaf pans. Bake for two hours. Let stand in pans 10 minutes before removing.

LUNCH

CHICKEN ALA SCHEER

1 cup cream	1/2 green bell pepper, chopped
1 tbsp. vegetable paste	1/2 red bell pepper, chopped
3 egg yolks, beaten	1/2 tsp. vegetable salt
2 cups cooked chicken, diced	1/2 tsp. paprika
2 egg yolks, hard boiled	1 tsp. wheat germ

166

In double boiler, make sauce by combining cream, vegetable paste and beaten egg yolks. Add remaining other ingredients and heat thoroughly. Serves 2-4.

DINNER

LEEK QUICHE

3 eggs	1/4 tsp. lemon pepper
1/4 cup half and half	juice of 1/2 lemon
1/4 tsp. brewer's yeast	1/4 cup grated swiss cheese
1 medium leek, chopped	1 whole wheat pie crust
1/4 tsp. nutmeg	

In medium bowl, beat eggs. Add half and half and mix well. Add yeast, leek, nutmeg, pepper, lemon juice and grated cheese. Blend well and pour into pie crust. Bake at 325 degrees 20 minutes or until top is brown and egg is set in center of pie.

CHAPTER 75
Smoking

The next time you're tempted to light up in a restaurant, remember they haven't caught the guy who calls himself the Deranged Douser. His solution to air pollution is a water pistol filled with lighter fluid.

Nicotine is absolutely the most addictive substance known to man. And if you include all the chemicals they put in cigarettes these days, it's easily the most dangerous.

You need all the help you can get to quit smoking. Here's some to get you started.

BREAKFAST

CHICKEN NOODLE SOUP

1 quart chicken stock	1/2 cup fresh or frozen peas
2 carrots, sliced	1/2 cup chopped cooked chicken
1 onion, sliced	1/2 cup uncooked wheat noodles
1 stalk celery, chopped	sea salt
1 tbsp. chopped parsley	pepper

Heat stock. Add carrots, onion, celery and parsley. Simmer, covered, over low heat 20 minutes. Add peas, chicken and noodles. Cover and simmer 10 minutes or until noodles are cooked. Add water if needed. Add salt and pepper to taste. Serves four.

LUNCH

CHICKEN AND LEEKS

4 boneless chicken breasts, skinned and pounded	dash paprika
1/4 lb. leeks, chopped	1/4 tsp. sea salt

Cut chicken into 1/2 inch cubes and place in frying pan. Add salt, paprika and leeks and cover bottom of pan with 1/4 inch water. Stew chicken, turning often and adding water if necessary. Heat well before serving. Serves 2-4.

DINNER

SAVORY PUMPKIN RING

2 cups pumpkin puree	dash allspice
2 tbsp. vegetable oil	1/2 tsp. sea salt
1 small onion, finely chopped	2 tsp. honey
1 small stalk celery with leaves, finely chopped	
3/4 cup fresh whole wheat bread crumbs	2 eggs, beaten
1/4 cup wheat germ	1/4 cup milk

Put pumpkin puree in large bowl. Oil one-quart ring mold and preheat oven to 350 degrees. Heat oil and saute onion and celery until just clear. Add bread crumbs and saute to mix well. Add mixture to pumpkin and blend. Add wheat germ, allspice, salt and honey. Mix well. Blend eggs and milk together. Add to pumpkin mixture. Pour puree into ring mold. Set mold in pan of hot water and bake about 45 minutes or until set. Unmold onto warm plate. Serves 6-8.

CHAPTER 76
Stress

"If the grass is greener in the other person's yard, let him worry about cutting it." - Fred Allen

For every minute you are angry, upset or frustrated, you lose 60 seconds of happiness. Most experts agree that allowing stress to take over your life will shorten it; not to mention create a pretty miserable one. But don't stress over the stress in your life.

Betcha didn't realize food can help you relax. Everybody's heard of warm milk to go to sleep. Well, milk, cheese and bananas are loaded with tryptophan, nature's sedative. So are whole grains and lean meat. So, when you feel stressed, or just need help with nerves, try some of these fine recipes.

BREAKFAST

PATIENCE POTATO SOUP

2 lbs. potatoes, chopped	dash white pepper
1 carrot, sliced	2 tsp. sea salt
2 leeks, sliced	4 cups milk
4 cups chicken or vegetable stock	

In large pot, cook all ingredients, except milk, for 25 minutes. Puree in blender or food processor. Add milk. Serve hot or cold.

LUNCH

MEATLESS BURGERS

burgers:

1 tsp. Savorex or Vegex	1 cup millet
1/4 cup hot water	2 tbsp. chopped black olives
1 cup grated raw potatoes	1 tbsp. wheat germ
1 cup oatmeal	1/8 tsp. sage
1/2 cup finely chopped onion	1 tsp. garlic salt

170

1/4 cup finely chopped macadamia nuts
1/3 cup finely chopped celery
1 sprig parsley, chopped

1 tsp. no-MSG soy sauce
1/4 tsp. sea salt

whole wheat pita bread

sauce:

1 cup yogurt
1/4 tsp. cayenne
2 tbsp. lemon juice

1 small tomato, chopped
1/2 cucumber, chopped
sea salt

In large bowl, dissolve Savorex in hot water. Mix with rest of ingredients and form patties. If batter is too thick, add more water. Saute in hot oil or broil until both sides are browned. To make sauce, combine all ingredients. Serve in whole wheat pita bread with sauce on top.

DINNER

NEW POTATO SOUFFLE

1 lb. new potatoes, steamed
1/2 tsp. brewer's yeast
1/4 tsp. nutmeg
1/4 tsp. black pepper

1/4 tsp. oregano
1/4 tsp. cold butter
1/4 cup grated cheddar cheese

Cut potatoes into thin slices and place in buttered shallow baking pan. Over the top sprinkle: brewer's yeast, nutmeg, pepper, oregano, cheese and bits of cold crumbled butter. Bake in 350 degree oven for 15 minutes or until tender and golden brown.

CHAPTER 77
Stretch Marks

On one of my many airline flights, I heard a lady ask the flight attendant where her seat was. I guess she was a regular flyer because the attendant replied "three inches lower than last year."

Gravity, pregnancy and extreme weight loss can cause stretch marks, on some people, and not on others. Why? Why do some people get them and others don't? The most important factor is the condition of their skin. With proper nutrition and exercise, skin is strong, supple and elastic. It will spring back into shape even after the expansion of pregnancy. To keep your skin in tip top shape, try these recipes.

BREAKFAST

PUMPKIN PIE IN GRANOLA CRUST

crust:
- 1-1/2 cup granola
- 1 cup almonds
- 1-1/2 cup shredded coconut
- 1/4 cup whole wheat flour
- 1/4 cup wheat germ
- 1 tsp. vanilla
- 1/2 - 2/3 cup skim milk or water

filling:
- 1-1/2 cup pumpkin
- 2 tbsp. honey
- 1/4 cup date sugar
- 3 tbsp. arrowroot
- 1/4 tsp. sea salt
- 1/2 cup skim milk
- 1/2 tsp. vanilla
- 1/2 tsp. lemon peel
- 1 tsp. ground coriander

To make crust, mix granola and almonds in blender until fine. Combine granola mixture with rest of ingredients and press into 9" pie pan. Bake 350 degrees 8-10 minutes or until lightly browned.

Combine filling ingredients in saucepan. Cook until thick, stirring occasionally. Put into blender and mix until smooth. Pour into baked pie crust. Refrigerate before serving.

LUNCH

CHICKEN CARIBE

2 tbsp. vegetable oil
1 3-4 lb. chicken, cut up
1 large onion, chopped
3 tomatoes, peeled, seeded and chopped
1 green bell pepper, seeded and chopped
1 clove garlic, chopped

1 tsp. sea salt
1/2 tsp. cumin
1/4 tsp. pepper
1 cup chicken stock
2 tbsp. whole wheat flour

Heat oil in skillet and brown chicken, a few pieces at a time. Place browned chicken in large pot or slow cooker. Add onions, tomatoes, bell pepper, garlic, salt, cumin, pepper and stock. Cover and simmer 45 minutes or cook in slow cooker on low for six hours. Remove chicken to warm platter. Mix 1/3 cup of cooking liquid into flour. Stir flour mixture into simmering pot until thick. Pour over chicken. Serves 4-6.

DINNER

PUMPKIN KARL

2 lbs. pumpkin, cut into sticks
1/2 cup honey
1/2 tsp. butterscotch flavoring

1/2 tsp. black pepper
several mint leaves
juice of 1/2 lemon

Combine honey, butterscotch flavoring, black pepper, mint leaves and lemon juice in a saucepan. Mix well and add pumpkin pieces. Cover pan and simmer 15 to 20 minutes.

CHAPTER 78
Teeth Grinding

Have you ever dreamed you were losing your teeth? That they were getting loose and falling out? Well, this nightmare is possible if you grind your teeth. Dentists warn their patients when they see telltale signs such as irregular and chipped edges: "Stop grinding your teeth!" as though it were a conscious act. There are even gizmos people wear at night, when they are most likely to do it, that lock the jaws together.

All this may be unnecessary, researchers have found, because deficiencies of calcium and pantothenic acid, a B vitamin, may in some cases be responsible. No need for a psychiatrist to uncover those deep-seated stresses, just eat foods high in these nutrients, like those contained in these recipes.

BREAKFAST

BULGUR PILAF

2 tbsp. sunflower oil	2 cups chicken or vegetable stock
1 onion, finely chopped	1 tsp. sea salt (optional)
1 cup bulgur	

Heat oil in heavy pot. Add onions and cook until onions are clear. Add bulgur; stir to coat grains with oil. Add stock and salt, if you wish. Bring to a boil. Cover, lower heat and simmer until liquid has been absorbed, about 15 minutes.

LUNCH

SOUTHWESTERN CHICKEN SALAD

1 cup cooked chopped chicken breast	1 tbsp. yogurt
1/8 cup sliced green onions	1/2 cup hot or mild red salsa
1/2 cup peeled jicama, cut into 1/2 inch cubes	
1 tbsp. chopped, fresh cilantro	3 green lettuce leaves, chopped
1/4 cup chopped tomato	grated lowfat cheese

174

In medium bowl, combine chicken, green onions, jicama, cilantro and tomato. In small bowl, combine yogurt and salsa. Add to chicken mixture and blend well. Spoon over lettuce and garnish with cheese.

DINNER

SPINACH SALAD

1 lb. green spinach	1/4 lb. grapes
1 carrot	1/4 lb. almonds, blanched
1/4 cup chopped cilantro or parsley	1 stalk celery
1/4 apple, diced	1/4 cup raspberry vinegar

Clean spinach, and slice carrots into very small pieces. Toss all ingredients together and serve.

CHAPTER 79
Tooth Decay

Did you hear about the latest diet? It's called the cavity diet. You can't eat anything that has holes in it.

Actually, it is possible to avoid tooth decay by eating certain foods. Foods that cause cavities are those high in starch and/or sugar and stick obstinately to the teeth. Other foods do the opposite and are credited with cleaning teeth: olives, nuts, especially cashews and yogurt.

BREAKFAST

NUTTY FRENCH TOAST

3/4 cup water
1/2 cup chopped cashews
4 chopped, pitted dates

pinch sea salt
whole wheat bread

Mix water, cashews, dates and salt in blender or food processor. Dip bread in mixture. Place on cookie sheet and brown both sides under broiler. Top with pureed plums, sugar-free jam or fresh fruit.

LUNCH

EGGPLANT GARREL

2 medium eggplants
2 medium tomatoes, sliced
1 medium onion, sliced
1/2 cup olives
1 clove garlic, chopped
1/8 tsp. oregano
1/8 tsp rosemary

1/4 tsp. parsley
1/2 tsp. parmesan cheese
1/4 tsp. black pepper
1/4 tsp. white pepper
1 tbsp. sliced almonds
2 tbsp. cold butter

Peel and slice eggplants into thin slices. Place in buttered 13" x 9" baking pan. Top with tomato slices, sliced onions, olives and garlic. Add oregano, rosemary, parsley, parmesan cheese, and black and white pepper. Add almond slices on top and a few crumbles of cold butter. Brown in oven (350 degrees) and serve.

DINNER

CASHEW-DRESSED SLAW

1 small head cabbage, finely shredded
1 cup fresh pineapple chunks
1 cup cashews, ground
1/4 cup water

1/4 cup honey
2 tbsp. cider vinegar
kelp

Place cabbage and pineapple in large salad bowl. Mix ground cashews in water to make a stiff paste. Add honey, vinegar and kelp to taste.   Pour over cabbage and pineapple. Toss. Best if marinated several hours prior to serving. Serves four.

CHAPTER 80
High Thyroid Function
(hyperthyroidism)

He who is stretched like a rubber band will soon find himself shooting for the moon.

The symptoms of an overactive thyroid gland: extreme perspiration, sleeplessness and jittery nerves mimic that of a long-term vitamin C and E deficiency, which eventually causes the thyroid to produce more hormone. Both disorders can be alleviated by adequate amounts of these vitamins. Other nutrients help restore the system to its proper balance. To get your balancing act together, try these recipes.

BREAKFAST

NUT LOAF

1 cup grated carrots	1 cup tomatoes
1/2 cup chopped parsley	1/2 cup chopped green bell pepper
1 clove garlic, chopped (optional)	2 tbsp. vegetable oil
2 cups chopped nuts	1/2 tsp. dill

Blend all ingredients in blender or food processor. Pack into oiled 8" x 4" loaf pan. Bake in 350 degree oven 45 minutes or until desired doneness. Serves 6.

LUNCH

EGGPLANT ASPARAGUS

2 medium eggplants	1/8 tsp. black pepper
1 bunch asparagus	1 tsp. chopped cilantro
1 cup half and half	2 tbsp. mozzarella cheese
1 tsp. nutmeg	2 tbsp. pinenuts

Peel eggplant and cut into french fry-size pieces. Cut asparagus in same lengths. Mix half and half, nutmeg, black pepper and cilantro. Pour into a buttered deep baking pan and add eggplant and asparagus. Top with cheese and pinenuts. Cook in 350 degree oven until browned and serve.

DINNER

CABBAGE SALAD

1 medium cabbage, grated	1/2 cup honey
1 clove garlic, chopped	1/4 cup raisins
1/4 tsp. black pepper	1/4 cup sunflower seeds
1/2 apple, sliced	1/2 cup white wine vinegar
1 onion, sliced	1/2 cup sour cream

In large bowl combine cabbage and garlic, black pepper, apple slices, onion slices, honey, raisins and sunflower seeds. Add white wine vinegar. Mix well. Let marinate several hours. Add sour cream just before serving.

CHAPTER 81
Low Thyroid Function
(hypothyroidism)

"Here is the test to find whether your mission on earth is finished: If you're alive, it isn't." - Richard Bach

If you are wondering why you have so many of the afflictions discussed in this book, it may be here that you should be looking. An under-active thyroid gland can produce a number of symptoms; from cold hands and feet to constipation, to an inability to think clearly. A reliable do-it-yourself test is found in my book *Foods That Heal.*

Healthy eating is essential to a healthy thyroid. These nutrient-packed recipes contain foods rich in iodine, the most important nutrient to an under-productive thyroid.

BREAKFAST

ASPARAGUS SOUP

1 lb. asparagus	1/8 tsp. nutmeg
2 quarts vegetable stock	1/8 tsp basil
2 leeks, chopped	1/8 tsp. oregano
2 onions, chopped	1/8 tsp. tarragon
2 carrots, chopped	1/8 tsp. marjoram
1 clove garlic, pressed	1/8 tsp. kelp
1 tsp. black pepper	chopped cilantro

In large pot combine all ingredients. Simmer over low heat until carrots are tender. Add cilantro on top just before serving.

LUNCH

FAVORITE BROILED FISH

6 fish filets	1 tsp. sea salt
2/3 cup toasted wheat germ	2 tbsp. lemon juice
1 tsp. paprika	2 tbsp. olive oil

1/2 tsp. chopped garlic
dash pepper

4-5 large mushrooms, sliced

Preheat broiler and oil shallow baking pan. Mix together wheat germ, paprika, garlic, pepper and salt. Roll filets in mixture to coat and place in baking pan. Mix lemon juice with oil and sprinkle over fish. Broil three minutes then turn filets over. Sprinkle on any remaining wheat germ mixture, add mushrooms and broil 3-5 minutes or until desired doneness.

DINNER

COLORFUL COLESLAW

1 lb. cabbage, grated
1 tart apple, grated
1 bell pepper, grated
1 carrot, grated

1 tsp. kelp
2 tbsp. mayonnaise
1 tbsp. lemon juice

Combine cabbage, apple, pepper, carrot and kelp. Mix well. Add mayonnaise and lemon juice. Blend thoroughly. Serves 4-6.

CHAPTER 82
Ulcers

"The more you try to avoid suffering, the more you suffer because smaller things. begin to torture you in proportion to your fear of suffering." Thomas Merton

If ulcers are your sore spot, relax and try these recipes. The foods contained in them condition the skin, and, in the case of intestinal ulcers, actually soothe inflamed tissues. They'll work on your hemorrhoids too!

BREAKFAST

MILLET SALAD

12 oz. millet	several dried mint leaves
1/4 cup chopped cilantro	1 cup white wine vinegar
1/2 medium yellow onion, chopped	1/2 tsp. black pepper
2 cloves garlic, chopped	1/4 tsp. cayenne pepper
1/4 tart green apple, chopped	2 tsp. chopped parsley
2 tbsp. chopped walnuts	

Steam millet and mix well with other ingredients, reserving 1 tbsp. walnuts and parsley for the top as a garnish.

LUNCH

CHARD-KASHA ROLLS

8-10 oz. chard leaves	1 large onion, chopped
6-1/2 cups boiling water	2 tsp. kelp
1 cup kasha	sea salt
1/2 cup dried split peas	pepper
1 tbsp. olive oil	2 cups sauerkraut

Wash chard leaves well. Drop them into boiling water until just limp. Remove leaves and reserve water. Rinse leaves in cold water and drain. Heat five cups of reserved water to boiling. Stir in kasha and peas. Simmer over low heat, covered,

20 minutes or until thick and fairly dry. Meanwhile, trim stems from chard leaves and lower half of the heavy center rib. Chop stem and rib fine. Set aside. Place cooked kasha and peas in large bowl. Heat oil in skillet and saute onion until just beginning to brown. Stir in kasha mixture. Add kelp and salt and pepper to taste.

Working with one chard leaf at a time, place 2-3 tablespoons of kasha mixture near the top edge of leaf. Roll leaf to enclose filling. Fill all leaves. (Reserve any leftover filling for a delicious and hearty breakfast.) Place half the sauerkraut and chopped chard stems and ribs in a large cooking pot. Top with chard rolls then remaining sauerkraut. Add one cup of the reserved water. Bring to a boil, cover and simmer over low heat 10 minutes to reduce liquid. Serves 6-8.

DINNER

ZUCCHINI SALAD

3-4 small zucchini, finely chopped	1/4 tsp. oregano
3 green onions, finely chopped	1 cup yogurt
2 tbsp. fresh chopped dillweed	1 tbsp. lemon juice
1 tbsp. chopped parsley	1 tsp. honey

In a large salad bowl toss together zucchini, green onion, dillweed, parsley and oregano. In small bowl, combine yogurt, lemon juice and honey. Pour over zucchini mixture and toss to mix well. Refrigerate 30 minutes or longer before serving. Serves 2-4.

CHAPTER 83
Water Retention

Before I caught on to the spirit of healthful eating, I had problems every month with water retention. The only solution it seemed, was to join Sea World as its main attraction.

Water retention, edema, or swelling, can be caused by allergies and nutritional deficiencies. And there are foods that actually work to expel retained water like cucumber, dill and asparagus. I've compiled recipes here that contain these vital nutrients and helpful foods so you won't feel like the largest mammal on earth.

BREAKFAST

CUCUMBER APPLE SALAD

2 large apples, thinly sliced
1 tsp. lemon juice
1 cucumber, seeded and thinly sliced
1/2 red onion, thinly sliced
2 oranges, segmented
3 tbsp. finely chopped parsley

1/4 cup rice vinegar
1/4 cup olive oil
1 tsp. ground cumin
pinch cayenne
1/2 cup sliced black olives

In large bowl combine apple and lemon juice. Add cucumber, onion, oranges and parsley. Combine vinegar, olive oil, cumin and cayenne; add to apple mixture and toss well. Garnish with black olives, if desired.

LUNCH

JERUSALEM ARTICHOKE SOUP

1 lb. Jerusalem artichokes, sliced
1 large onion, chopped
2 stalks celery with leaves, chopped
4 cups water

1 tsp. dill seed
1/2 cup packed fresh sorrel leaves
1/4 cup lemon juice

Put all ingredients, except lemon juice, into large pot. Bring to boil. Lower heat and simmer 25 minutes. Let soup cool. Puree in blender or food processor. Add lemon juice. Serve hot or cold. Serves 4-6.

DINNER

ASPARAGUS SALAD

1 lb. asparagus	1/4 tsp. black pepper
1/2 cup tarragon vinegar	1/4 tsp. lemon pepper
1/2 yellow onion, sliced	1/4 tsp. Tabasco sauce

Steam asparagus, let cool, and place on a platter. Mix all remaining ingredients together, mixing well, and pour over asparagus.

CHAPTER 84
Wrinkles

"If God had to give a woman wrinkles, He might have at least put them on the soles of her feet." - Ninon de Lenclos (1620-1705)

The newest thing under the sun is health warnings against being under the sun, although you don't have to be a genius to figure it out when you look at the grizzled, lined faces of farmers who spend their days tending crops.

Wrinkles aren't a necessary sign of age. They can be prevented and even reversed! With a healthy, whole foods diet rich in fiber, nutrients, and plenty of water and exercise, the only place you'll see channels and furrows is in the garden.

BREAKFAST

JEWELED RICE PILAF

2 tbsp. oil	1/4 cup currants or raisins
1/3 cup chopped onion	3 cups boiling water
1/4 cup sunflower seeds	sea salt
1 cup brown rice	pepper
1/3 cup chopped apricots	

Heat oil in large pot and saute onion until soft. Add sunflower seeds and rice. Cook about two minutes more, stirring. Stir in apricots and currants or raisins. Add boiling water and return to a boil. Cover and simmer 40 minutes or until rice is done. Season to taste with salt and pepper. Serves six.

LUNCH

ORANGE TURKEY SALAD

2 oranges	1/2 tsp. curry powder
3 cups diced cooked turkey	1/2 cup mayonnaise
1 cup chopped celery	1/2 cup toasted slivered almonds

1 cup seedless green grapes   lettuce leaves
1/2 tsp. sea salt

Peel and section oranges over bowl to reserve two tablespoons juice. Combine
turkey, celery, grapes, orange sections, juice and salt. Cover and refrigerate one
hour. Combine curry and mayonnaise. Blend thoroughly. Add to turkey mixture
and toss to coat evenly. Serve on lettuce leaves and topped with almonds. Serves
8-10.

DINNER

SILKY SKIN SALAD

2 medium apples, diced   1/4 cup yogurt
1 cup chopped celery   1/2 tsp. Dijon mustard
1 cup seedless grapes   1/2 cup chopped walnuts
2 tbsp. lemon juice

Toss the apples, celery and grapes together with lemon juice. Mix yogurt and
mustard together; toss with apple mixture. Sprinkle in walnuts. Serves six.

God be with Ye

Until we meet again in the pages of another book, I want to say goodbye to you. The word goodbye is a fascinating one. It originated from the contraction of the expression "God be with ye."

Along with a nutritious menu for the body, it is necessary to have the proper ingredients to make up your emotional and spiritual menu for greater health and well-being.

The Bible passages you are about to read have been such a blessing to me, I wanted to share them with you, my new found friends.

"A merry heart doeth good like a medicine, but a broken spirit drieth the bones." Proverbs 17:22

"Trust in the Lord with all thy heart; and lean not unto thine own understanding." Proverbs 3:5

"Delight thyself also in the Lord, and he shall give thee the desires of thine heart." Psalms 37:4

Now that you have met my book, *The Light at the End of the Refrigerator*, you have made a new friend. If you wish to make more, read my other books: *Foods That Heal, The Diet Bible* and *Nutrition - The Cancer Answer.*

INDEX

NUTRITION
The Cancer Answer
by Maureen Salaman

Voted the Best Health Book
by the American Book Exchange
A Perennial Best Seller in its 9th Printing

In the time it takes for you to read this, hundreds of Americans will have died of cancer. These deaths could have been prevented if the American public and the orthodox medical establishment had only been aware of the information in this book.

NUTRITION: THE CANCER ANSWER presents, in understandable detail, the discoveries and cancer prevention information contained in the National Academy of Science report, together with practical advice to apply these logical principles of nutrition to your life NOW, not 20 years from now.

Most of the 365,000 Americans who will become cancer victims this year could have remained cancer free, or at least controlled the disease, with the information contained in this book.

NUTRITION: THE CANCER ANSWER is a result of 12 years of vigorous research by Maureen Salaman, well-known author in the field of health and cancer prevention.

NUTRITION: THE CANCER ANSWER will:

- Give you research-based proof that cancer can be prevented and controlled.

- Rid you of the fear of ever contracting cancer in your lifetime.

- Present carefully researched studies of various societies which enjoy cancer-free lives.

- Show how you can enjoy exuberant good health untouched by the "one in three" cancer epidemic. Included is a Gourmet Guide to cancer prevention filled with easy and delicious recipes for vibrant good health.

NUTRITION: THE CANCER ANSWER, 309 pages

Suggested retail price: $14.95 + $3.50 shipping

Quantity Discounts Available

Customary Discounts to Trade Book Buyers

Order from:
M.K.S., Inc.
1259 El Camino Real, Ste.1500
Menlo Park, CA 94025
(415) 854-9355
FAX: 415-854-9292

THE DIET BIBLE
by Maureen Salaman

In the introduction of this book, Maureen confesses how she played pendulum, swinging from normal weight to overweight and back.

UNTIL

She discovered simple bible principles that enabled her to formulate a wonder-working diet.

Learn what others now know: the secret to her weight-watching success.

Her simple regimen features foods that melts away un-wanted pounds.

THE DIET BIBLE, 304 pages

Retail price: $17.50 + $3.50 shipping and handling

Order today from:
M.K.S., Inc.
1259 El Camino Real, Ste. 1500
Menlo Park, CA 94025
(415) 854-9355
FAX: 415-854-9292

MAUREEN KENNEDY SALAMAN
"A Speaker of Attraction"

Maureen Kennedy Salaman is a unique combination of talents and capabilities that have impacted the readers of her books, articles, plus her tapes, television appearances and live audiences around the world.

She is not only an award-winning writer, but a speaker of extraordinary ability. Maureen has shared the wisdom, wit and insight of her health and motivational messages at over one thousand engagements over the last two decades in over 300 cities around the country and around the world!

As a dynamic performer, she communicates a totally positive approach to health and problem solving, and helps listeners program their lives with strategies for healthful and successful living.

She is in touch with the wellness challenges confronting people every day. Most importantly, she is able to share, through research, experience and ancedotes, what works, what doesn't and why.

She has the unique ability to hold an audience's attention for an hour or an entire day by involving the group with the questions which they are most concerned. She covers a wide variety of action-oriented presentations, ranging from "Conquering Cravings," to "Correcting Hair Loss" to "Breaking the Bondage of Addiction."

Her special annointing is in communicating her totally positive approach to Christian audiences. The secular and business world respect her as a communicator of extraordinary ability.

To bring Maureen Salaman's life-enhancing message to your church, or company, or to order her books, tapes or newsletter contact:

M.K.S., Inc.
1259 El Camino Real, Ste. 1500
Menlo Park, CA 94025
(415) 854-9355
FAX: 415-854-9292